Springer
Tokyo
Berlin
Heidelberg
New York
Hong Kong
London
Milan
Paris

K. Nakamura, Y. Toyama, Y. Hoshino (Eds.)

Cervical Laminoplasty

With 105 Figures

Springer

Kozo Nakamura, M.D., Ph.D.
Professor and Director, Department of Orthopaedic Surgery, Faculty of Medicine
The University of Tokyo
7-3-1 Hongo, Bunkyo-ku, Tokyo 113-0033, Japan

Yoshiaki Toyama, M.D., Ph.D.
Professor and Chairman, Department of Orthopaedic Surgery, School of Medicine
Keio University
35 Shinanomachi, Shinjuku-ku, Tokyo 160-8582, Japan

Yuichi Hoshino, M.D., Ph.D.
Professor and Director, Department of Orthopaedic Surgery
Jichi Medical School
3311-1 Yakushiji, Minamikawachi-machi, Kawachi-gun, Tochigi 329-0498, Japan

ISBN 4-431-70304-7 Springer-Verlag Tokyo Berlin Heidelberg New York

Library of Congress Cataloging-in-Publication Data applied for.

Printed on acid-free paper

Typesetting: SNP Best-set Typesetter Ltd., Hong Kong

SPIN: 10786454

Preface

When, in 1960, ossification of the posterior longitudinal ligament (OPLL) was clearly recognized as a disease, the level of interest in cervical spine surgery increased remarkably in Japan. Results of subsequent studies confirmed that there were certain clinical disadvantages associated with laminectomy, including postoperative kyphosis and rapid development of OPLL. Owing to technical limitations associated with anterior decompression surgery, there was an urgent need to develop surgical procedures based on a posterior approach.

Professor Susumu Hattori at Yamaguchi University reported just such a break-through technique in 1970. Without this revolutionary technique, subsequent surgical advances would not have been possible, and those doctors who followed Professor Hattori are truly indebted to his contribution. In the next 10 years, until 1980, many new surgical techniques were introduced, and it is these techniques that are discussed in this book. During this time, our mentors, Professor Kiyoshi Hirabayashi at Keio University and Professor Takahide Kurokawa at the University of Tokyo, introduced the open-door technique and the spinous process-splitting technique, respectively. Both procedures are still widely performed today. Looking back, this 10-year period was a wonderful decade in which many dreams were realized.

In the 20 years that followed, the characteristics, advantages, and disadvantages of each surgical technique have been analyzed and compared, and procedures modified. No marked differences have been found among the various techniques, and each surgeon has his or her favorite procedure. Some studies have also followed patients for almost 20 postoperative years, and various laminoplasty techniques have been shown to provide favorable clinical outcomes.

Despite such positive results, however, laminoplasty is performed mainly in Japan, and there seems to be a misconception among surgeons in other countries that this surgical technique is specialized and difficult. Although there have been some reports on laminoplasty in the English literature, we believe the amount of information obtainable from these articles is insufficient to perform the procedure. We therefore decided to publish this book as a guide for surgeons who want to learn about laminoplasty and to help them to perform this surgery safely and effectively. Successful laminoplasty requires a certain amount of knowledge and skill, and it should not be performed based on limited data.

It is our sincerest wish that this book will assist surgeons to perform laminoplasties safely, knowing that there are various techniques available, that each technique has its own advantages and disadvantages, and that aftercare plays an important role. The Publication of *Cervical Laminoplasty* is a source of great pride for us, and we will be very pleased indeed if this book proves useful to readers.

June 2003

Kozo Nakamura
Yoshiaki Toyama
Yuichi Hoshino

Contents

Contributors

Aita, Ikuo (p. 119)
Department of Orthopaedic Surgery, Institute of Clinical Medicine, University of Tsukuba, Tennohdai 1-1-1, Tsukuba, Ibaraki 305-8575, Japan

Akamaru, Tomoyuki (p. 127)
Department of Orthopaedic Surgery, School of Medicine, Kanazawa University, 13-1 Takara-machi, Kanazawa 920-8641, Japan

Chiba, Kazuhiro (pp. 27, 139, 163)
Department of Orthopaedic Surgery, School of Medicine, Keio University, 35 Shinanomachi, Shinjuku-ku, Tokyo 160-8582, Japan

Echigoya, Naoki (p. 111)
Department of Orthopedic Surgery, Hirosaki University, 5 Zaifu-cho, Hirosaki 036-8562, Japan

Goto, Sumio (p. 65)
Department of Orthopaedic Surgery, National Center of Neurology and Psychiatry, Kohnodai Hospital, 1-7-1 Kohnodai, Ichikawa, Chiba 272-8516, Japan

Harata, Seiko (p. 111)
Department of Orthopedic Surgery, Hirosaki University, 5 Zaifu-cho, Hirosaki 036-8562, Japan

Hirabayashi, Kiyoshi (p. 27)
Department of Orthopaedic Surgery, School of Medicine, Keio University, 35 Shinanomachi, Shinjuku-ku, Tokyo 160-8582, Japan

Hirabayashi, Shigeru (pp. 99, 153)
Department of Orthopaedic Surgery, Saitama Medical Center, Saitama Medical School, 1981 Tsujido, Kamoda, Kawagoe, Saitama 350-8550, Japan

Hoshino, Yuichi (pp. 15, 169)
Department of Orthopaedic Surgery, Jichi Medical School, 3311-1 Yakushiji, Minamikawachi-machi, Kawachi-gun, Tochigi 329-0498, Japan

Ishizuka, Kyoko (pp. 99, 153)
Department of Orthopaedic Surgery, Saitama Medical Center, Saitama Medical School, 1981 Tsujido, Kamoda, Kawagoe, Saitama 350-8550, Japan

Iwasaki, Hiroaki (p. 83)
Orthopaedic Surgery, Hattori Memorial Hospital, 4244 Kammaki, Kitakatsuragi, Nara 639-0200, Japan

Iwasaki, Motoshige (p. 47)
Department of Orthopaedic Surgery, Faculty of Medicine, The University of Tokyo, 7-3-1 Hongo, Bunkyo-ku, Tokyo 113-0033, Japan

Kato, Yoshiharu (p. 75)
Department of Orthopaedic Surgery, Tokyo Women's Medical University, 8-1 Kawada-cho, Shinjuku-ku, Tokyo 162-8666, Japan

Kawahara, Norio (p. 127)
Department of Orthopaedic Surgery, School of Medicine, Kanazawa University, 13-1 Takara-machi, Kanazawa 920-8641, Japan

Kiya, Tetsuro (p. 175)
Department of Orthopaedic Surgery, Koshigaya Hospital, School of Medicine, Dokkyo University, 2-1-50 Minami-Koshigaya, Koshigaya, Saitama 343-8555, Japan

Kobayashi, Tadayoshi (p. 127)
Department of Orthopaedic Surgery, School of Medicine, Kanazawa University, 13-1 Takara-machi, Kanazawa 920-8641, Japan

Maruiwa, Hirofumi (pp. 27, 163)
Department of Orthopaedic Surgery, School of Medicine, Keio University, 35 Shinanomachi, Shinjuku-ku, Tokyo 160-8582, Japan

Matsumoto, Morio (pp. 27, 139, 163)
Department of Orthopaedic Surgery, School of Medicine, Keio University, 35 Shinanomachi, Shinjuku-ku, Tokyo 160-8582, Japan

Moriya, Hideshige (p. 65)
Department of Orthopaedic Surgery, Chiba University School of Medicine, Chiba 260–8670, Japan

Murakami, Hideki (p. 127)
Department of Orthopaedic Surgery, School of Medicine, Kanazawa University, 13-1 Takara-machi, Kanazawa 920-8641, Japan

Nakamura, Kozo (pp. 3, 47)
Department of Orthopaedic Surgery, Faculty of Medicine, The University of Tokyo, 7-3-1 Hongo, Bunkyo-ku, Tokyo 113-0033, Japan

Nanbu, Koshi (p. 127)
Department of Orthopaedic Surgery, School of Medicine, Kanazawa University, 13-1 Takara-machi, Kanazawa 920-8641, Japan

Nohara, Yutaka (p. 175)
Department of Orthopaedic Surgery, Koshigaya Hospital, School of Medicine, Dokkyo University, 2-1-50 Minami-Koshigaya, Koshigaya, Saitama 343-8555, Japan

Okada, Akihiro (p. 111)
Department of Orthopedic Surgery, Hirosaki University, 5 Zaifu-cho, Hirosaki 036-8562, Japan

Saiki, Kunio (pp. 99, 153)
Department of Orthopaedic Surgery, Saitama Medical Center, Saitama Medical School, 1981 Tsujido, Kamoda, Kawagoe, Saitama 350-8550, Japan

Saita, Kazuo (p. 169)
Department of Orthopaedic Surgery, Jichi Medical School, 3311-1 Yakushiji, Minamikawachi-machi, Kawachi-gun, Tochigi 329-0498, Japan

Seichi, Atsushi (pp. 3, 47)
Department of Orthopaedic Surgery, Faculty of Medicine, The University of Tokyo, 7-3-1 Hongo, Bunkyo-ku, Tokyo 113-0033, Japan

Tomita, Katsuro (p. 127)
Department of Orthopaedic Surgery, School of Medicine, Kanazawa University, 13-1 Takara-machi, Kanazawa 920-8641, Japan

Toyama, Yoshiaki (pp. 27, 139, 163, 185)
Department of Orthopaedic Surgery, School of Medicine, Keio University, 35 Shinanomachi, Shinjuku-ku, Tokyo 160-8582, Japan

Tsuzuki, Nobuyuki (pp. 99, 153)
Department of Orthopaedic Surgery, Saitama Medical Center, Saitama Medical School, 1981 Tsujido, Kamoda, Kawagoe, Saitama 350-8550, Japan

Ueda, Yurito (p. 83)
Department of Orthopaedic Surgery, Nara Medical University, 840 Shijo-cho, Kashihara, Nara 634-8522, Japan

Ueyama, Kazumasa (p. 111)
Department of Orthopedic Surgery, Hirosaki University, 5 Zaifu-cho, Hirosaki 036-8562, Japan

Wadano, Yasuyoshi (p. 119)
Department of Orthopaedics, Center for Medical Sciences, Ibaraki Prefectural University of Health Science, 4669-2 Ami-machi, Inashiki-gun, Ibaraki 300-0394, Japan

Yabuki, Takeshi (p. 119)
Yabuki Orthopaedic Clinic, 2-12-18 Keyakidai, Moriya, Ibaraki 302-0128, Japan

Yamazaki, Masashi (p. 65)
Department of Orthopaedic Surgery, Chiba University School of Medicine, Chiba 260–8670, Japan

Yokoyama, Toru (p. 111)
Department of Orthopedic Surgery, Hirosaki University, 5 Zaifu-cho, Hirosaki 036-8562, Japan

Part 1
History

History of Laminoplasty

Kozo Nakamura and Atsushi Seichi

Cervical laminoplasty was developed in Japan in the early 1970s to resolve postoperative problems after conventional laminectomy for instability and deformity which caused a recurrence of myelopathy; there have since been many modifications. The aim of laminoplasty is to expand the spinal canal, to preserve the posterior structure of the cervical spine and assure stability, and to prevent the formation of a postlaminectomy membrane. In this chapter, we describe the background to the development of laminoplasty for cervical stenotic myelopathy.

Laminectomy of the Cervical Spine

Posterior approaches for the removal of agents compressing the spinal cord were reported between the sixteenth and eighteenth centuries [1], and laminectomy for intraspinal tumors was first performed in the nineteenth century [1]. In the early twentieth century, cervical spondylosis began to be recognized as a cause of cervical myelopathy. Cervical spondylosis as a cause of cord compression was first understood by Mixter and Barr [1, 2]. In 1956, Clarke and Robinson [1, 3] advocated that cervical spondylotic myelopathy be defined as a distinct clinical entity. Studies on the pathophysiology of cervical spondylotic myelopathy continued [4], but it was not until the late 1950s that operative techniques through the posterior approach were described for the treatment of cervical spondylosis. The report by Yuhl et al. [5] on 32 cases of cervical spondylotic myelopathy treated with wide laminectomy and a section of the dentate ligament with the removal of any accessible anterior bony spurs showed this was very unsatisfactory. Clarke and Robinson [3] described four types of laminectomy: laminectomy alone, laminectomy with opening of the dura for inspection and subsequent closure, laminectomy with a section of dentate ligaments, and laminectomy with the removal of disc material. None of them showed satisfactory results.

Department of Orthopaedic Surgery, Faculty of Medicine, The University of Tokyo, 7-3-1 Hongo, Bunkyo-ku, Tokyo 113-0033, Japan

Mayfield [6] abandoned extradural curettage of the bony spurs through the posterior approach and adopted a wide laminectomy combined with multiple-level foraminotomies. The short-term results were better, but some of the patients developed cervical subluxations and late progressive spondylosis. The results of laminectomy were universally unsuccessful [7, 8]. These unsatisfactiry results forced spinal surgeons to search for alternatives.

Anterior Cervical Surgery

An anterior approach to the cervical spine was described by Smith and Robinson [9, 10]. They stated that the anterior procedure had less morbidity than laminectomy combined with foraminal decompression posteriorly, and allowed safer removal of a degenerated disc without disturbing the spinal cord. In the United States and Europe, technical advances in anterior cervical spine surgery continued. Cloward [11] used the method of trephine drill and dowel interposition grafting. As the surgical results of anterior surgery for cervical spondylosis improved [12, 13], the anterior procedure was adopted as the first option, while the posterior approach by laminectomy was viewed as having a risk of instability, an inability to prevent progression of the condition. A multiple-segment anterior fusion technique, as described by Bailey and Badgley [14, 15], has also been used successfully. When the cervical spine is kyphotic, the best surgical option has been believed to be the anterior approach [16]. When combined with halo vests, even four-level cervical corpectomy has been available. Recently, a system employing several kinds of locking plates has been used to prevent graft dislodgement. A freeze-dried allograft has been used to achieve anterior fusion. One stage of cervical anterior decompression and posterior stabilization has become another option. However, the problems associated with multiple-level anterior fusion still include not only graft dislodgement and pseudoarthrosis, but also accelerated degenerative changes above and below the fusion [17].

Development of Laminoplasty

In contrast to the development of anterior cervical surgery in the United States and Europe, the posterior procedure advanced in Japan with the development of the high-speed drill. The main causes of cervical myelopathy in Japanese patients have been multilevel spinal cord compression due to multilevel spondylosis with developmental spinal canal stenosis, or multilevel ossification of the posterior longitudinal ligament (OPLL). These conditions have caused Japanese spinal surgeons to choose a posterior procedure as a treatment option. Kirita and co-workers [18, 19] have used simultaneous decompressive laminectomy since 1968, and their results showed dramatic improvements compared with the previously reported results of laminectomy. The decompressive procedure has become safer with the use of an air-drill rather than a rongeur. However, several authors reported that extensive laminectomy sometimes caused postoperative instability, including swan neck deformity [20–24]. How to preserve the structural mechanics of the posterior cervical spine has also been a problem.

Expansive Z-laminoplasty, which was the first type of laminoplasty, was developed by Oyama and Hattori in 1972 [25]. The aim of this procedure was to prevent postoperative invasion of the laminectomy membrane, which was believed to be one factor causing late deterioration following surgery. In this method, the spinous processes are excised and the laminae are thinned using an air-drill. After making a Z-shaped incision of the laminae, the spinal canal is enlarged, while bony protection of the spinal cord is retained (see the chapter by S. Kawai in this volume). This technique has been employed mainly in Yamaguchi University, Yamaguchi, Japan, but has not become popular because of its technical complexity. Hirabayashi et al. [26] devised the simpler technique of expansive open-door laminoplasty of the unilateral hinge type in 1977 (see the chapter by K. Chiba in this volume). The mid- and long-term results are reliable from the standpoint of neurological maintenance, preventing postoperative kyphotic deformity, and preventing the progression of OPLL [27–29]. In the 1980s, preliminary reports of certain types of cervical laminoplasty appeared and the results were generally judged to be satisfactory. Itoh and Tsuji [30] added a further refinement to Hirabayashi's method for stabilizing lifted lamina using a bone block, which was called "en bloc laminoplasty" (see the chapter by Y. Katoh in this volume). Kurokawa et al. [31] developed double-door laminoplasty (spinous-process-splitting laminoplasty) in 1980. In their original procedure, small bone blocks from the posterior iliac crest were grafted to keep the split spinous processes separated (see the chapter by A. Seichi in this volume). Except for Hattori's Z-shaped laminoplasty and Ohmori's method (suspension laminotomy [32]), laminoplasty of the cervical spine falls into two categories according to the design of the osteotomy: the unilateral hinge-type method such as Hirabayashi's, and the bilateral hinge-type method such as Kurokawa's. Variations of the unilateral hinge-type method include Itoh's method (en bloc laminoplasty), the Yamagata University method (see the chapter by M. Hayashi in this volume), and the Chiba University method (see the chapter by H. Moriya in this volume). Matsuzaki et al. [33] added unilateral fusion to Hirabayashi's method. Variations of the bilateral hinge-type method of laminoplasty include the techniques of Iwasaki and Yabuki. Iwasaki et al. [34] reported the results of open-door laminoplasty, with removal of spinous processes and thinning down of the lamina (see the chapter by H. Iwasaki in this volume) in 1982. In 1982, Yabuki began double-door laminoplasty using spinous processes as bone blocks (see the chapter by I. Aita in this volume).

Recently, in procedures using iliac bone blocks such as Kurokawa's method, an artificial spacer has often been used rather than an autograft in order to decrease the operation time and to avoid postoperative pain around the donor graft site [35–37] (see the chapter by S. Harata in this volume).

As cervical laminoplasty has become popular in Japan, Japanese spinal surgeons have shown on interest not only in osseous reconstruction, but also in reconstruction of the soft tissues. The reattachment of the erector spinae muscles to C2 and preservation of the continuity of the nuchal ligament have been recognized as important in preventing flexion deformity [38–40] (see the chapter by Y. Hoshino in this volume). Various modifications of laminoplasty to preserve the posterior elements of the cervical spine, and the anatomical reconstruction of these elements as far as possible, also have been reported [41, 42]. However, it is not yet clear to what degree stability is improved and motion of the cervical spine is preserved with the preservation and reconstruction of the posterior soft tissues.

Some workers have reported a reduction in the range of motion (ROM) as a disadvantage after laminoplasty [43, 44], and postoperative maintenance of the ROM of the neck remains a problem. Early mobilization of the neck has recently been recommended in order to avoid postoperative stiffness [41, 43]. On the other hand, some workers are of the opinion that this reduction of the ROM may be beneficial in maintaining neurological improvements and may suppress the growth of OPLL [28, 29, 44].

The reliable long-term results of laminoplasty have recently caused spinal surgeons to discuss an extension of the surgical indication for cervical stenotic myelopathy. Are patients with a very mild disability due to cervical stenosis candidates for laminoplasty instead of conservative treatment? Is laminoplasty a better treatment option for elderly people than laminectomy in spite of the longer operative time? These questions must be addressed and decisions made in the near future.

Laminoplasty Versus Laminectomy

The results of cervical laminectomy were poor in the early period, and several authors reported spinal deformity, instability, and the formation of hematoma in the dead space following surgery [20, 21, 24, 45–48]. However, there is still a general opinion that cervical laminectomy is one of the viable options for multilevel spondylosis and OPLL, especially for aged patients when the anterior approach is not favorable, because the high-speed air-drill has made this procedure safer and the technique is now simple [49, 50]. There are also several reports about attempts to prevent postlaminectomy instability by posterior fusion with or without instrumentation, instead of laminoplasty [24, 51]. Posterior instrumentation surgery includes correction of any malalignment of the cervical spine. With regard to post-operative instability after laminectomy, there are reports that cervical laminectomy in which the facets are not disturbed can be well tolerated [52, 53], and that deformity occurs more frequently in children than in adults [46, 54–56]. Raynor et al. [52], in biomechanical studies of the cervical segments in human cadavers, demonstrated that shear strength is not compromised until more than 50% of the facets have been removed bilaterally. Some surgeons insist that postoperative instability after laminectomy does not occur unless the facet joints are sacrificed [45, 53, 57].

There is no prospective control study to confirm the superiority of laminoplasty over laminectomy, and such claims thus remain controversial. However, the long-term results of laminoplasty are stable from the point of view of neurological recovery and prevention of deformity [27, 43]. Moreover, the technique of laminoplasty is safer and simpler than inexperienced spinal surgeons often imagine, and the risk of intraoperative bleeding is minimal because the surgeon need not enter the posterolateral epidural space in which the rich venous plexus exists. Therefore, most spinal surgeons who are familiar with laminoplasty have abandoned the use of laminectomy.

Laminoplasty Versus Anterior Decompression

The controversy over laminoplasty versus subtotal corpectomy for multiple cervical spondylosis remains unresolved [16, 58, 59]. Laminoplasty is frequently chosen as a surgical option for Japanese patients because their cervical canal is generally narrower than that of American and European individuals, and multi-segmental OPLL is a common cause of cervical myelopathy. In contrast to the situation in Japan, the predominant pathology of cervical myelopathy has been believed to be anterior in Europe and the United States, and anterior decompression and stabilization has been viewed as a radical treatment for cervical spondylotic myelopathy because anterior surgery removes all of the anterior spinal compression and does not allow motion at the pathological segments. Laminoplasty is seen as having an indirect decompression effect resulting from a posterior shift of the spinal cord without removing anterior pathological structures such as discs and spurs. However, since buckling of the ligamentum flavum in the posterior spinal canal is one main causative factor in cervical myelopathy, and preexisting cervical spinal stenosis is another, laminoplasty can be considered to have a direct decompression effect on the spinal cord because it removes the posterior pathological structures. Stenosis in the adjacent levels after anterior decompression and fusion is believed to be a long-term complication which makes myelopathy worse, especially in patients with congenital spinal stenosis. In contrast, laminoplasty involves total widening of the cervical canal and makes a long-standion decompressing effect possible. The pathophysiology of cervical spondylotic myelopathy involves static factors which directly compress the spinal cord, as well as dynamic factors caused by movement of the cervical spine. Anterior spinal fusion is effective in removing the dynamic factors, but laminoplasty also has a restrictive effect on the spine since it reduces the cervical range of motion through arthrosis of the facet joints. The indications for laminoplasty for myelopathy with cervical kyphosis have not been established. The surgical effect of laminoplasty for patients with severe cervical kyphosis is unclear, but our experience has shown this procedure to be effective for those with mild cervical kyphosis [43]. Differences regarding the choice of optimal surgical decompression for multi-level compressive myelopathy still persist.

References

1. Dunn EJ, Seybold EA (1998) The development of surgical approaches for cervical radiculopathy and spondylotic myelopathy. In: Ono K, Dvorák J, Dunn E (ed) Cervical spondylosis and similar disorders. World Scientific, Singapore, pp 357–394
2. Mixter JW, Barr JS (1934) Rupture of the intervertebral disc with involvement of the spinal canal. N Engl J Med 211:210–215
3. Clarke E, Robinson PK (1956) Cervical myelopathy. A complication of cervical spondylosis. Brain 79:483–510
4. Robinson RA, Afeche N, Dunn E, et al. (1977) Cervical spondylotic myelopathy. Etiology and treatment concepts. Spine 2:89–99
5. Yuhl ET, Duke H, Rasmussen T, et al. (1955) Diagnosis and surgical therapy of chronic midline cervical disc protrusion. Neurology 5:494–509
6. Mayfield FH (1965) Cervical spondylosis: a comparison of anterior and posterior approaches. Clin Neurosurg 13:181–188
7. Symon L, Lavender P (1967) The surgical treatment of cervical spondylotic myelopathy. Neurology 17:117–126
8. Nurick S (1972) The natural history and the results of surgical treatment of the spinal cord disorder associated with cervical spondylosis. Brain 95:101–105
9. Robinson RA, Smith G (1955) Anterolateral cervical disc removal and interbody fusion for cervical disc syndrome. Bull Johns Hopkins Med J 96:223–224
10. Smith GW, Robinson RA (1958) The treatment of certain cervical spine disorders by the anterior removal of the intervertebral disc and interbody fusion. J Bone Joint Surg 40A:607–624
11. Cloward RB (1958) The anterior approach for removal of ruptured cervical discs. J Neurosurg 15:602–614

12. Bohlman H (1977) Cervical spondylosis with moderate to severe myelopathy. A report of 17 cases treated by Robinson. Anterior cervical discectomy and fusion. Spine 2:151–162
13. Concha S, McQueen JD (1977) Anterior cervical fusions for spondylotic myelopathy. Spine 2:147–150
14. Yang K, Lu X, Cai Q, et al. (1987) Cervical spondylotic myelopathy treated by anterior multi-level decompression and fusion. Clin Orthop Rel Res 221:161–164
15. Bailey RW, Badgley CE (1960) Stabilization of the cervical spine by anterior fusion. J Bone Joint Surg 42A:1372–1383
16. Hirabayashi K, Bohlman HH (1995) Multiple cervical spondylosis. Laminoplasty versus anterior decompression. Spine 20:1732–1734
17. Baba H, Furusawa N, Imura S, et al. (1993) Late radiographic findings after anterior cervical fusion for spondylotic myeloradiculopathy. Spine 18:2167–2173
18. Kirita Y, Miyazaki K, Lin T, et al. (1975) Posterior decompression in myelopathy due to ossification of the posterior longitudinal ligament (in Japanese). Rinsho Seikeigeka 10:1077–1085
19. Miyazaki K, Kirita Y (1983) Extensive simultaneous multisegmental laminectomy for myelopathy due to the ossification of the posterior longitudinal ligament in the cervical spine. Spine 11:531–542
20. Mikawa Y, Shikata J, Yamamuro T (1987) Spinal deformity and instability after multilevel cervical laminectomy. Spine 3:6–11
21. Sim FH, Suien HJ, Bickel WH, et al. (1974) Swan-neck deformity following extensive cervical laminectomy. J Bone Joint Surg 56A:564–580
22. Ishida Y, Suzuki K, Ohmori K, et al. (1989) Critical analysis of extensive cervical laminectomy. Neurosurgery 24:215–222
23. Yonenobu K, Okada K, Fuji T, et al. (1986) Causes of neurologic deterioration following surgical treatment of cervical myelopathy. Spine 11:818–823
24. Miyazaki K, Tada K, Matsuda Y, et al. (1989) Posterior extensive simultaneous multisegmental decompression with posterolateral fusion for cervical myelopathy with cervical instability and kyphotic and/or S-shaped deformities. Spine 14:1161–1170
25. Kawai S, Sunago K, Doi M, et al. (1988) Cervical laminoplasty (Hattori's method). Procedure and follow-up results. Spine 13:1245–1250
26. Hirabayashi K, Watanabe K, Wakano K, et al. (1983) Expansive open-door laminoplasty for cervical spinal stenotic myelopathy. Spine 8:693–699
27. Satomi K, Nishi Y, Kohno T, et al. (1994) Long-term follow-up studies of open-door expansive laminoplasty for cervical stenotic myelopathy. Spine 19:507–510
28. Hirabayashi K, Satomi K (1988) Operative procedure and results of expansive open-door laminoplasty. Spine 13:870–876
29. Hirabayashi K, Miyakawa J, Satomi K, et al. (1981) Operative results and postoperative progression of ossification among patients with ossification of cervical posterior longitudinal ligaments. Spine 6:354–364
30. Itoh T, Tsuji H (1985) Technical improvement and results of laminoplasty for compressive myelopathy in the cervical spine. Spine 10:729–736
31. Kurokawa T, Tsuyama N, Tanaka H, et al. (1982) Enlargement of the spinal canal by the sagittal splitting of the spinous process (in Japanese). Bessatsu Seikeigeka 2:234–240
32. Ohmori K, Ishida Y, Suzuki K (1987) Suspension laminotomy: a new surgical technique for compression myelopathy. Neurosurgery 21:950–957
33. Matsuzaki H, Toriyama S, Sugawara T, et al. (1982) Cervical canal-expansive laminoplasty with unilateral fusion (in Japanese). Bessatsu Seikeigeka 2:249–252

34. Iwasaki H, Yokota H, Ishii M, et al. (1982) Expansive laminoplasty (in Japanese). Bessatsu Seikeigeka (Orthop Surg) 2:228–233
35. Hase H, Watanabe T, Hirasawa Y, et al. (1991) Bilateral open laminoplasty using ceramic laminas for cervical myelopathy. Spine 1991:1269–1276
36. Hirabayashi S, Kumano K (1999) Contact of hydroxy spacers with split spinous processes in double-door laminoplasty for cervical myelopathy. J Orthop Sci 4:264–268
37. Nakano K, Harata S, Suetsuna F, et al. (1992) Spinous process-splitting laminoplasty using hydroxyapatite spinous process spacer. Spine 17:S41–43
38. Sasai K, Saito T, Akagi I, et al. (2000) Cervical curvature after laminoplasty for spondylotic myelopathy. Involvement of yellow ligament, semispinalis cerviis muscles, and nuchal ligament. J Spinal Disord 13:26–30
39. Kurokawa T, Nakamura K, Hoshino Y (1995) On double-door laminoplasty splitting spinous processes for stenosis of the cervical spine (in Japanese). Rinsho Seikeigeka 30:566–571
40. Hirabayashi K (1995) Expansive open-door laminoplasty. In: Sherk HH (ed): The cervical spine. An atlas of surgical procedures. Lippincott, Philadelphia, pp 233–250
41. Tsuzuki N, Abe R, Saiki K, et al. (1996) Tension-band laminoplasty of the cervical spine. Int Orthop 20:275–284
42. Yoshida M, Otani K, Shibasaki K, et al. (1992) Expansive laminoplasty with reattachment of spinous process and extensor musculature for cervical myelopathy. Spine 17: 491–497
43. Seichi A, Takeshita K, Nakamura K, et al. (2001) Long-term results of double-door laminoplasty for cervical stenotic myelopathy. Spine 26:479–487
44. Baba H, Maezawa Y, Furusawa N, et al. (1995) Flexibility and alignment of cervical spine after laminoplasty for spondylotic myelopathy. Int Orthop 19:116–121
45. Butler JC, Whitecloud TD (1992) Postlaminectomy kyphosis. Causes and surgical management. Orthop Clin North Am 23:505–511
46. Kamioka Y, Yamamoto H, Tani T, et al. (1989) Postoperative instability of cervical OPLL and cervical radiculomyelopathy. Spine 14:1177–1183
47. Herkowitz H (1988) A comparison of anterior cervical fusion, cervical laminectomy, and cervical laminoplasty for the surgical management of multiple-level spondylotic radiculopathy. Spine 13:774–780
48. Albert T, Vacarro A (1998) Postlaminectomy kyphosis. Spine 23:2738–2745
49. Raynor RB (1998) Laminectomy for cervical spondylosis: indications and techniques. In: Ono K, Dvorak J, Dunn E (ed) Cervical spondylosis and similar disorders. World Scientific, Singapore, pp 477–499
50. Epstein J, Epstein N (1994) Laminectomy for spondylotic myelopathy and radiculopathy. In: Sherk HH (ed) The cervical spine. An atlas of surgical procedures. Lippincott, Philadelphia, pp 219–232
51. Callahan R, Johnson R, Margolis R, et al. (1977) Cervical facet fusion for control of instability following laminectomy. J Bone Joint Surg 59A:991–1002
52. Raynor RB, Pugh J, Shapiro I (1985) Cervical facetectomy and its effect on spine strength. J Neurosurg 63:278–282
53. Guigui P, Benoist M, Deburge A (1998) Spinal deformity and instability after multilevel cervical laminectomy for spondylotic myelopathy. Spine 23:440–447
54. Katsumi Y, Honma T, Nakamura T (1989) Analysis of cervical instability resulting from laminectomies for removal of spinal cord tumor. Spine 14:1171–1176
55. Catell S, Clark L (1967) Cervical kyphosis and instability following multiple laminectomies in children. J Bone Joint Surg 49A:713–720

56. Bell DF, Walker JL, O'Connor G, et al. (1994) Spinal deformity after multiple-level cervical laminectomy in children. Spine 19:406–411
57. Nowinski GP, Visarius H, Nolte LP, et al. (1993) A biomechanical comparison of cervical laminoplasty and cervical laminectomy with progressive facetectomy. Spine 14:1995–2004
58. Yonenobu K, Hosono N, Iwasaki M, et al. (1992) Laminoplasty versus subtotal corpectomy: a comparative study of results in multisegmental cervical spondylotic myelopathy. Spine 17:1281–1284
59. Herkowitz HN, Kurz LT, Overholt DP (1990) Surgical management of cervical soft disc herniation: a comparison between the anterior and posterior approach. Spine 15:1026–1030

Part 2

Surgical Anatomy

Anatomical Knowledge Required for Laminoplasty

YUICHI HOSHINO

In all four-legged animals, the extensors are dominant over the flexors in the neck in order to maintain the head in a horizontal position. In the human neck, the extensors are also dominant. A cross section of the human neck (Fig. 1) shows that 70% of the muscles present are posterior to the rotational axis of anteroposterior flexion movements.

In the human neck, the extensor power is about twice the flexor power (Table 1). Because the posterior muscles and their actions in the neck are important, surgeons should have a thorough anatomical knowledge of the nuchal muscles when carrying out laminoplasty by a posterior approach.

In laminoplasty, the spinal process, lamina, and facet joint are exposed, and osteoplasty is performed using instruments such as a high-speed drill. Therefore, the morphology of the bone tissue in the posterior spinal area should also be well understood.

Nuchal Muscles and Ligaments

Nuchal Ligament

The nuchal ligament is present in the shallowest median area. This ligament forms a septum between the right and left trapezius muscles. It is attached to the external occipital protuberance on the rostral side, and becomes the supraspinous ligament at the 6th or 7th spinal process on the caudal side. In cattle with a heavy head, the nuchal ligament is more than 10 mm thick even in calves, and is considered to play a role in limiting the neck flexion, and increasing the efficiency of the extensors in the neck. Therefore, great case should be taken not to interrupt the continuity of this ligament. In ossification of the spinal ligaments, ossification also occurs in the nuchal ligament, and is observed as Barsony's sign on plain X-ray films.

Department of Orthopaedic Surgery, Jichi Medical School, 3311-1 Yakushiji, Minamikawachi-machi, Kawachi-gun, Tochigi 329-0498, Japan

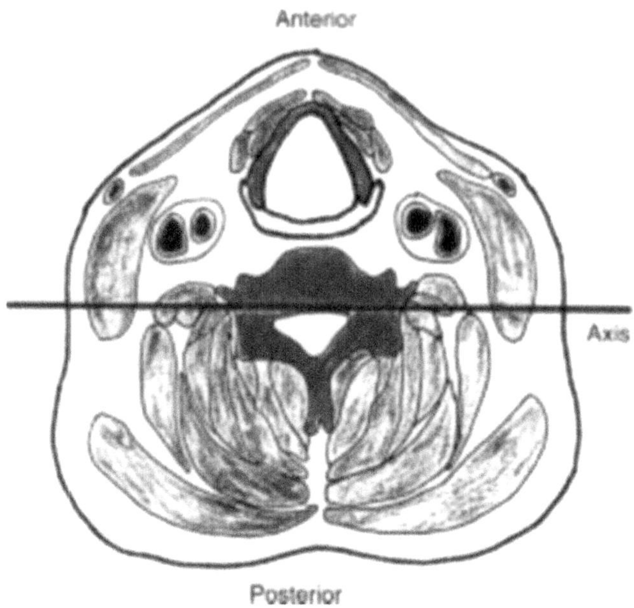

Fig. 1. A cross section of the human neck. More than 70% of the muscles present are posterior to the rotational axis of anterior–posterior flexion movements

Table 1. Neck muscle power in 39 normal volunteers, 30 males and 9 females mean age 30 years

	Extension	Flexion
Males	281 ± 39 N	134 ± 27 N
Females	167 ± 23	60 ± 13

Shallow Nuchal Muscles

The trapezius and splenius capitis muscles are present in the shallow layer. In a median approach, the trapezius muscles appear on the right and left sides of the nuchal ligament. When the trapezius muscle is incised, the site of the insertion of the splenius capitis muscle into the spinal process is exposed. The only way to maintain the continuity of the nuchal ligament described above is to transect the unilateral trapezius muscle from the nuchal ligament, and therefore a paramedian approach is used (Fig. 2). In this approach, the contralateral nuchal muscles are covered by the muscular septum, which minimizes any danger to them.

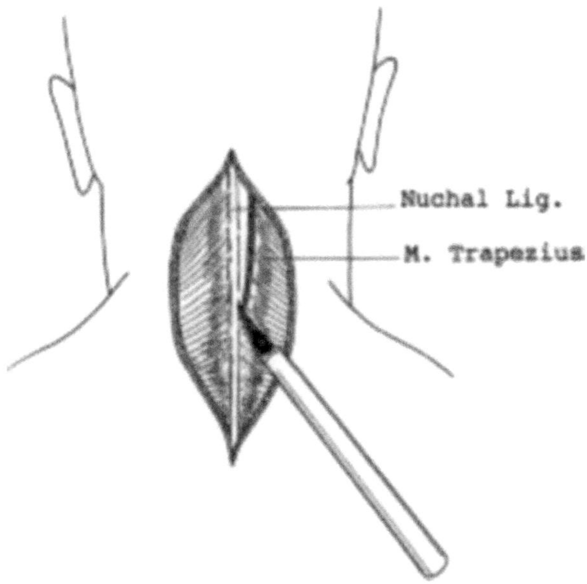

Fig. 2. Paramedian approach. Transection of the unilateral trapezius muscle from the nuchal ligament is the only way to restore its continuity.

Deep Nuchal Muscles

When the site of the insertion of the splenius capitis muscle into the spinal process at the lower cervical spine is dissected and retracted to the right and left, the interspinalis and semispinalis cervicis muscles appear. The semispinalis cervicis muscle originates in the C2 spinal process, which is readily palpated as a large osseous protrusion. The rectus capitis posterior major muscle and the inferior oblique muscle are attached to the rostral area of the C2 spinal process (Fig. 3). The semispinalis cervicis muscle is the largest of the extensors in the deep layer that are attached to the cervical spinal process. The C2 spinal process is probably large because of the attachment of these important extensors. After dissection of the muscles attached to the C2 spinal process, they usually shorten by about 2–3 cm as a result of muscle tension. It is therefore rational to restore them to their original place before skin closure in order to recover muscle tension (Fig. 4).

The small multifidus muscle is attached to the caudal margin of the lamina.

Supraspinous Ligament and Interspinous Ligament

These ligaments should be resected in the spinal-process splitting method, but a method to preserve them has also been devised (reference). The nuchal

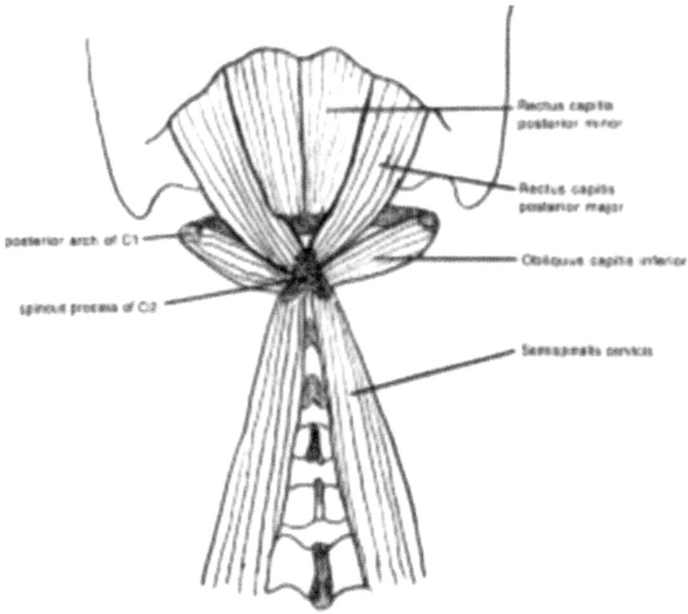

Fig. 3. Nuchal muscles in the deep layer. The spinal process of the axis has many attachments from many muscles, and this is the reason for its size.

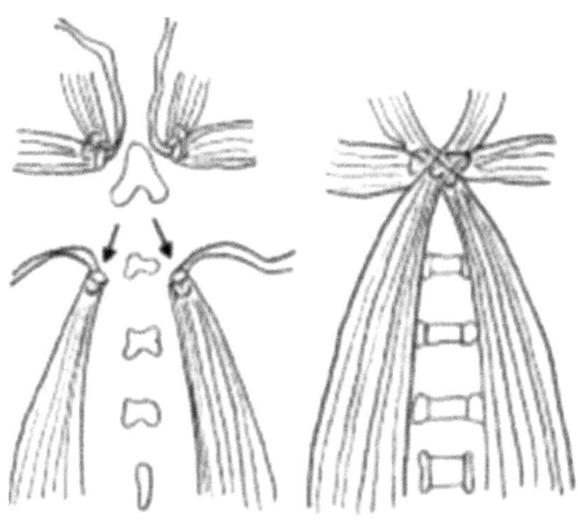

Fig. 4. Preservation of muscle tension before closing the wound. After the deep muscles are dissected from the C2 spinal process, they shrink by up to 2–3 cm (**a**). Therefore, before closing the wound it is necessary to pull the muscles into their original positions in order to preserve muscle tension (**b**)

ligament becomes the supraspinous ligament at the tip of the C7 spinal process, and is continuous with the thoracic spine.

Yellow Ligament

The yellow ligament connects the laminae and forms the posterior wall of the spinal canal. In the thoracic and lumbar spine, the yellow ligament is often ossified and compresses the spinal cord. In the cervical spine, ossification of the yellow ligament is very rarely observed. Calcification of the yellow ligament, which is an amorphous deposition of calculi, has been reported more frequently (Fig. 5).

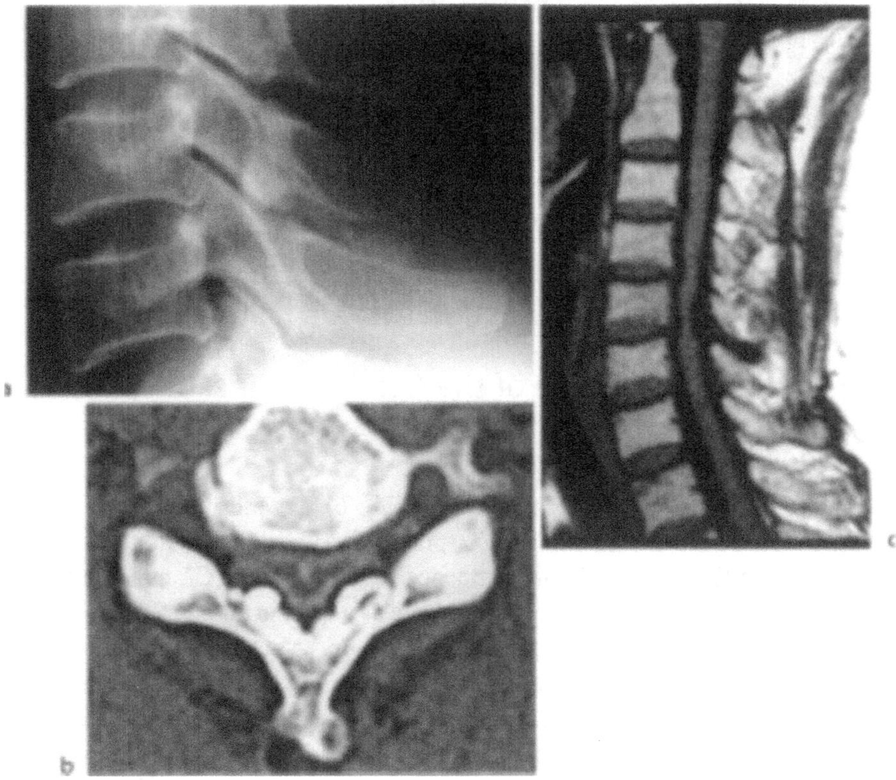

Fig. 5. Calcification of the yellow ligament in a 72-year-old woman with cervical myelopathy. **a** Plain film. A calcified mass can be observed between the C5/6 laminae and the spinal processes. **b** Computed tomography showed the calcified ligamentum flava compressing the spinal cord. **c** T1-weighted magnetic resonance image showing a low-signal area at the level of C5/6

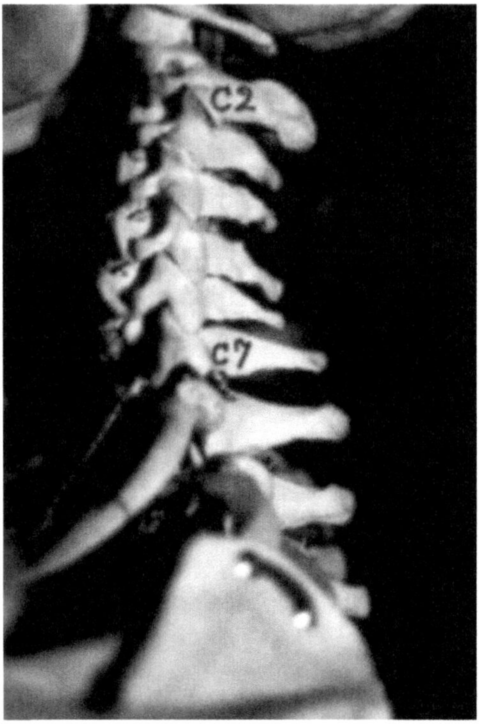

Fig. 6. Lateral view of the cervical spine. C2 and C7 have large spinal processes

Posterior Bone Tissue of the Cervical Spine

Spinal Process

The C2 and C7 spinal processes are large (Fig. 6). As described above, important muscles are attached to the C2 spinal process, while a firm nuchal ligament from the occipital bone is attached to the tip of the C7 spinal process. Each spinal process has an important role as a lever arm to extend the neck. In laminectomy by a conventional posterior approach, these spinal processes are resected, which causes postoperative instability and kyphosis. The original purpose of laminoplasty was to preserve osseous elements as the attachment sites of the muscles and ligaments in the posterior area of the cervical spine, and overcome problems observed after conventional laminectomy.

The atlas lacks the spinal process, and the muscles attached to the atlas are not large. Therefore, when decompression is necessary, many surgeons perform resection of the atlas alone. Since the C2 spinal process is large, and the lamina is thick, laminoplasty is relatively difficult. When a lateral gutter is made as a hinge, it is often very deep. Midline splitting is easy because of the adequate thickness of the spinal process. The C3–5 spinal processes often

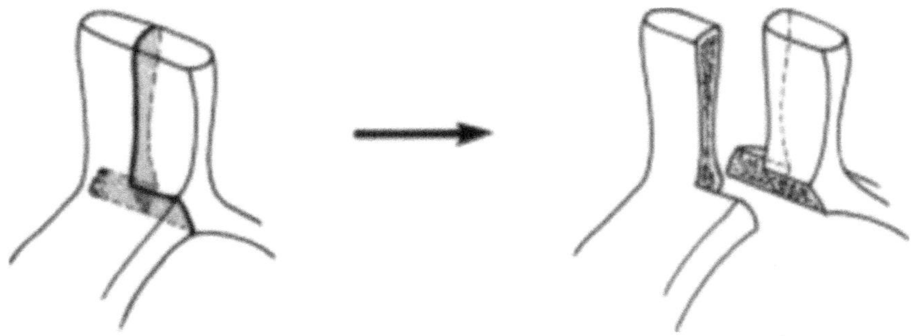

Fig. 7. A special method for splitting a thin spinal process, which is difficult to split without breakage

have a tip angled to the right or left, but the C6 and C7 spinal processes are plate-like. In people with less muscle, such as females, the spinal process is often thin, and midline splitting requires some special techniques (Fig. 7).

Lamina and Facet Joint

A lateral view of the lamina shows an inclination; the lamina is deeply set on the rostral side and less deeply on the caudal side. When the lamina is cut or transected, the rostral side becomes deeper. In laminoplasty, the area which is cut or transected is the medial margin of the facet joint, which corresponds to a horizontal part of the laminar inclination toward the lateral area. To avoid invasion of the facet joint, the site of this cut should be determined very carefully.

In spondylosis of the spine, the facet joint is often thickened, and identification of the location of the lateral gutter based on laminar morphology is difficult. The right and left widths of the spinal canal can be determined using computed tomography (CT) films.

Nerves

In the routine posterior midline approach in the neck, no important nerves are encountered. However, the C2 posterior branch of the greater occipital nerve has its dorsal root ganglion lateral to the lateral margin of the dura mater (Fig. 8), penetrates the M. semispinalis capitis, and runs cranially. To avoid damage to this nerve, the right and left retraction of the muscle layer should be limited to the width of the lateral margin of the facet joint.

The deep nuchal muscles are innervated by the posterior branch of the nerve root. This posterior branch passes the lateral margin of the facet joint

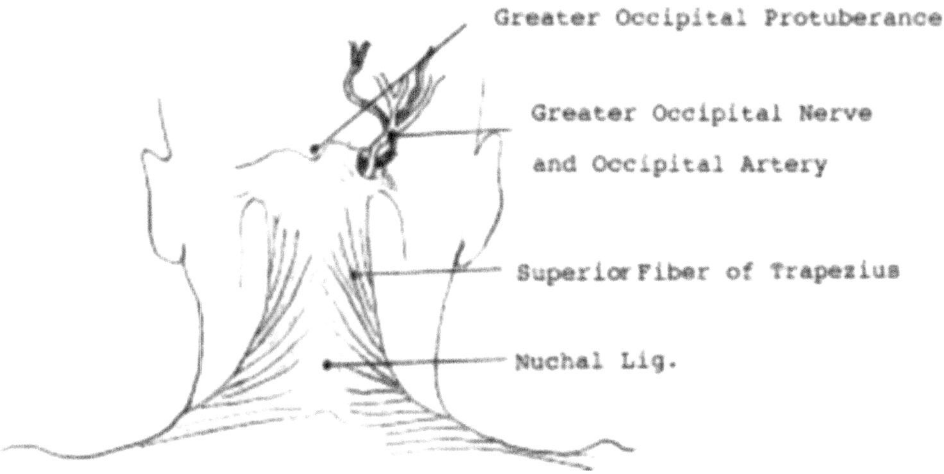

Fig. 8. The greater occipital nerve and occipital artery, which are bilateral to the greater occipital protuberance. When the wound exposure needs to be wide, they should be remembered and protected

and enters the dorsal muscle, which also limits the width of the right and left retraction of the muscle layer.

Blood Vessels

In the conventional cervical posterior median approach, major blood vessels are not encountered. However, in patients with athetoid-type cerebral palsy, the origin of muscles such as the M. semispinalis capitis is sometimes transected along the superior nuchal line of the cranial bone to reduce involuntary movements. In such cases, the occipital artery, which is two finger-breadths from the midline, should be taken into consideration.

In laminoplasty, the venous system presents problems. In particular, procedures to the upper cervical spine tend to cause massive bleeding. Between the posterior arch of the atlas and the lamina of the axis, there is the venous plexus called the longitudinal vertebral venous sinus (Fig. 9) on both sides, and great care is necessary when the C2 lateral gutter is cut. When this venous plexus is damaged, bleeding cannot be controlled with conventional hemostatic agents, and compression hemostasis for more than half an hour is required. This venous plexus should be protected from injury by the high-speed drill by using fine retractors.

The drainage veins from the lamina and spinal process run out of the bone via a small hole, and enter the deep nuchal muscles that are closely attached

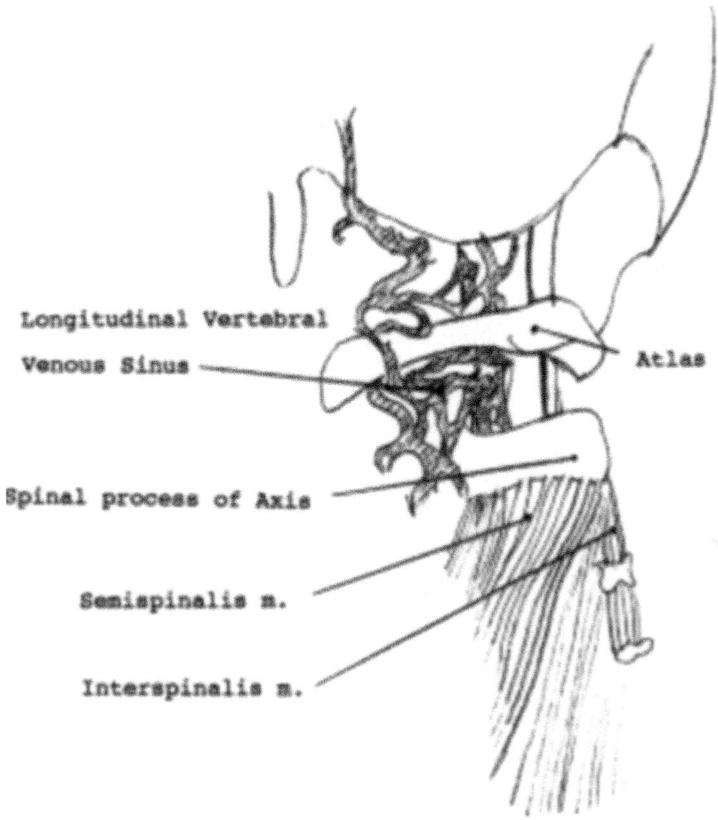

Fig. 9. Longitudinal vertebral venous sinus between the C1 and C2 laminae. If the operational procedure extends to the C2 lamina, the venous sinus between the C1 and C2 laminae often bleeds profusely. Therefore, the venous sinus must be protected from the high-speed drill

to the bone. These veins are transected in subperiosteal exposure of the lamina, and are recognized as bleeding spots. The bone hole should be treated with bone wax, and bleeding from the corresponding muscles should be completely controlled by electrocautery. If hemostasis is inadequate, bleeding will occur not only during, but also after the operation.

When the lamina is expanded, the venous plexus in the epidural cavity appears. This plexus is dense on the right and left sides of the spinal dura mater, but relatively coarse in the posterior median area. Therefore, when the inner cortex of the lamina is transected, the bleeding volume is relatively slight by the bilateral open method, which involves manipulation in the median area. However, the unilateral open method causes marked bleeding from the venous plexus on the open side of the spinal canal, and requires careful hemostasis manipulation.

The control of bleeding from the veins is very important in this surgical technique. To control the bleeding volume, anatomical knowledge of the venous system described above is essential. In addition, control of the venous pressure in the neck is also vital. If the operation is performed in the prone position, compression of the abdomen should be avoided by the correct use of a laminectomy table, and the venous pressure in the neck should be reduced by tilting the operating table in order to elevate the head area by 10–20°. These methods are useful for reducing bleeding.

Part 3

Basic Procedures

Expansive Open-Door Laminoplasty

Kazuhiro Chiba, Hirofumi Maruiwa, Morio Matsumoto, Kiyoshi Hirabayashi, and Yoshiaki Toyama

Introduction

Until 1968, when Kirita [1] devised a sophisticated technique for extensive laminectomy in which the laminae were thinned and divided at the midline with a high-speed drill, both patients and surgeons had suffered from unpredictable results with conventional laminectomy. Being both safe and effective, Kirita's technique brought remarkable progress in the surgical results of cervical compressive myelopathy. However, problems such as postoperative kyphosis, the vulnerability of the unprotected spinal cord, and the formation of a laminectomy membrane remained unsolved problems [2]. To address these problems, in 1973, Hattori and co-workers devised an expansive Z-laminoplasty in which the spinal canal was totally reconstructed with preservation of the posterior protective structures [3, 4]. However, this technique did not gain widespread acceptance because it was too technically demanding as well as time-consuming. Hirabayashi et al. [5] modified Kirita's method and decompressed the spinal cord by making bony gutters in both sides of the lamina followed by en-bloc resection of the laminae. The idea of open-door laminoplasty evolved when Hirabayashi [6] noted that pulsation of the dural tube occurred when he lifted one side of the laminae, indicating that sufficient decompression was obtained even before total resection of the laminae. He performed the first case of this procedure in 1977, and named it expansive open-door laminoplasty (ELAP; eelap). Since then, more than 500 patients have undergone this procedure at Keio University Hospital and affiliated hospitals with favorable results.

Although ELAP is not a radical decompression surgery that directly removes anterior pathological structures such as protruded discs and ossified ligaments, it has a total decompression effect induced by the dorsal shift

Department of Orthopaedic Surgery, School of Medicine, Keio University, 35 Shinanomachi, Shinjuku-ku, Tokyo 160-8582, Japan

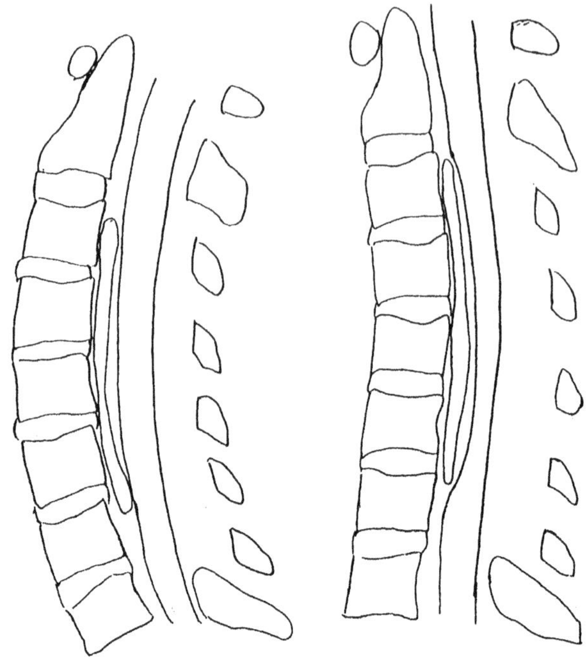

Fig. 1. Mechanism of decompression in Expansive Open-Door Laminoplasty (ELAP). Total decompression induced by the dorsal shift of the spinal cord is expected, in addition to local direct decompression in patients with lordosis (**a**). However, local decompression alone is effective in those with kyphosis (**b**)

of the spinal cord as long as patient's cervical alignment is maintained in lordosis, in addition to the local decompression effect of the displacement of the laminae directly relieving impingement on the spinal cord (Fig. 1) [7]. Several studies have confirmed that the decompression effect of ELAP is virtually equivalent to that of laminectomy and anterior decompression followed by fusion [8–10]. The incidence of instability, disc herniation, and spondylotic changes in the adjacent levels, which may lead to a salvage operation, was much lower after ELAP than after anterior decompression and fusion [5, 11].

The posterior structures, including the lamina and supra-and interspinous ligaments, are preserved, and the cervical muscles are reattached to reconstruct the spinal canal to maintain the preoperative cervical alignment, and at the same time to restore cervical stability [12]. Herkowitz [13] concluded from a biomechanical study that the stability of the cervical spine after ELAP was not significantly different from that of the intact spine. Kyphotic deformity or instability after ELAP that required salvage anterior correction and fusion has never been experienced in this clinic [5, 14].

Although a number of technical modifications, such as the use of bone grafts and spacers, have been made, this fundamental yet innovative technique forms the basis for all other procedures and remains the most viable choice for the surgical treatment of compressive myelopathy. When compared with other modified laminoplasties, ELAP is much simpler and safer, and has fewer surgical impacts, including a shorter operating time, less bleeding, and a lower incidence of complications [5, 10, 15, 16]. All these factors contribute to the widespread acceptance of ELAP, with increasing numbers of patients undergoing this procedure [5, 17].

Surgical Indications

Before the recognition of the concept of spinal stenosis, our indications for ELAP were based mainly on the extent of the pathology. If the spinal cord compression was confined within three segmental levels, anterior decompression followed by fusion was selected whereas ELAP was indicated for patients with a lesion extending beyond four segmental levels [18].

In accordance with the gradual acceptance of the concept of spinal stenosis, our surgical strategy has changed. Our retrospective long-term follow-up study on anterior cervical fusion revealed that degeneration in the adjacent levels of fusion progressed significantly in 85% of patients, and that subclinical compression of the dura was found in 65% of patients on follow-up magnetic resonance imaging (MRI). Moreover, revision surgeries were necessary in over 10% of the patients owing to the recurrence of myelopathy, and the majority of these patients had developmental spinal stenosis (anteroposterior [AP] diameter of the spinal canal under 13 mm on lateral neutral films) that was detected on a retrospective review of preoperative radiographs [19].

The presence of spinal canal stenosis has therefore become the determining factor when choosing a surgical option for patients with cervical myelopathy. The authors consider ELAP to be the treatment of choice for all patients with spinal canal stenosis whether the patient has single-level disc herniation, spondylosis, or segmental ossification of the posterior longitudinal ligaments (OPLL) [5, 20]. Even if patients have no spinal canal stenosis, if they have a multilevel lesion that extends beyond two segmental levels we prefer ELAP over anterior fusion. Recently, therefore, our indication for anterior cervical fusion for cervical myelopathy has been limited to patients having a single-level lesion without spinal canal stenosis [19]. When a patient has severe established kyphosis associated with spinal stenosis, we plan a two-stage surgery, which consists of first-stage ELAP followed by second-stage corrective anterior fusion. However, the secondary anterior fusion is usually unnecessary because a satisfactory improvement in the myelopathy can be obtained after the first-stage ELAP in the majority of such cases.

Our previous studies have revealed that the preoperative duration of myelopathy, the age of the patient at the time of surgery, a predisposition to trauma, and the severity of the spinal canal stenosis were factors that significantly affected the clinical results. Patients over 65 years of age, those with myelopathy of more than 2 years' duration, those with an onset of symptoms due to trauma, and those with severe spinal canal stenosis had significantly poor surgical results [14, 21, 22]. With respect to the timing of the surgery, we therefore recommend ELAP as early as possible before the spinal cord is irreversibly damaged, especially in relatively young and active patients with severe spinal canal stenosis even if they do not have severe myelopathy, to obtain better clinical outcomes [5]. ELAP is an ideal procedure that is considered reliable because it has the same decompression effect as laminectomy, it is considered much safer and easier than anterior fusion for a severely deteriorated spinal cord, and this safety and reliability are the keys that make early operation possible [23].

ELAP seems to be a rational procedure for typical cervical stenotic myelopathy, whereas other expansive laminoplasties that use bone grafting, spacers, or plates may be indicated for exceptional cases with a high degree of instability, such as cerebral palsy [5]. Although we have no experience of such cases, some investigators have even reported the efficacy of ELAP in patients with radiculopathy [8].

Procedures

Instruments Necessary for ELAP

The use of a high-speed drill is essential, and a small lamina spreader together with fine-tipped Kerrison rongeurs make the removal of the ligamentum flavum safe and easy (see Fig. 7). Otherwise, no other special surgical instruments are necessary, and ordinary instruments for cervical laminectomy are sufficient.

Positioning of the Patient

The patient is placed in a prone position on a surgical table on which sponge pads are placed to relieve excessive pressure on the shoulders and the iliac crests. The head is securely fixed with a Mayfield fixator that is firmly attached to the surgical table. Both knees are bent at a right angle and the lower legs are firmly fixed with shin supports attached perpendicular to the surgical table. Then the table is tilted cranially upward at an angle of approximately 30° to reduce venous congestion. The neck is flexed slightly forward

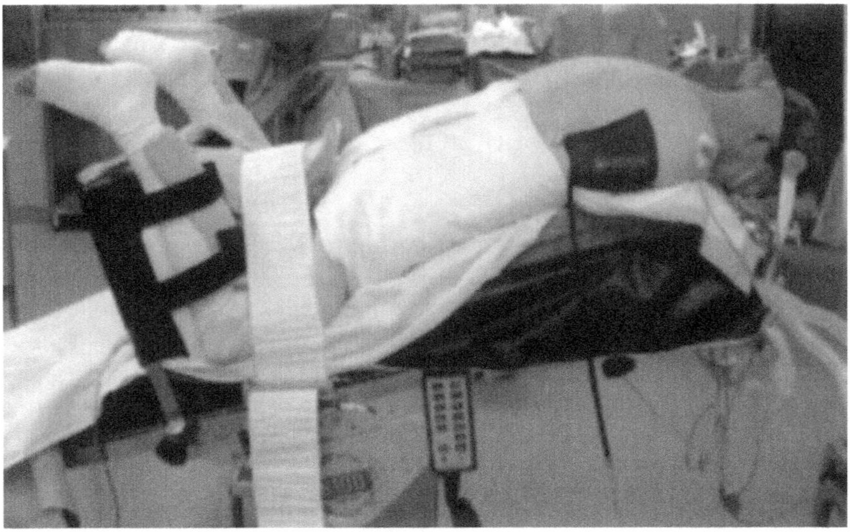

Fig. 2. Position of the patient

to open the interspinous spaces and to bring the posterior aspect of the neck to a horizontal plane (Fig. 2).

Techniques

Approach

The external occipital protuberance (inion), and the spinous processes of C2 and C7 serve as guides to the midline position (Fig. 3). Once a straight midline incision of the appropriate length has been made, follow the central plane along the nuchal ligament down to the spinous processes to avoid inadvertent bleeding. Retraction of the skin and subcutaneous tissues bilaterally with Gelpi or Adson retractors helps clarify the midline.

Lamina Exposure

Expose the tips of the spinous processes with a cautery, and then strip the bilateral paracervical muscles from the laminae, usually between C3 and C7, with a Cobb elevator and/or a cautery (Fig. 4). Care should be taken not to violate the supra-and interspinous ligaments and the facet joint capsules while detaching the paraspinal muscles from the laminae. We also preserve the attachment of the bilateral semispinalis cervicis muscles at the inferior tips of the C2 spinous process as much as possible, since these muscles are crucial for the maintenance of cervical lordosis. The tips of the long spinous processes of C6 and C7 are shortened to match the length of those of C3, C4, and C5 to avoid the closure of the laminar door by pressure from the paracervical muscles at wound closure (Fig. 5).

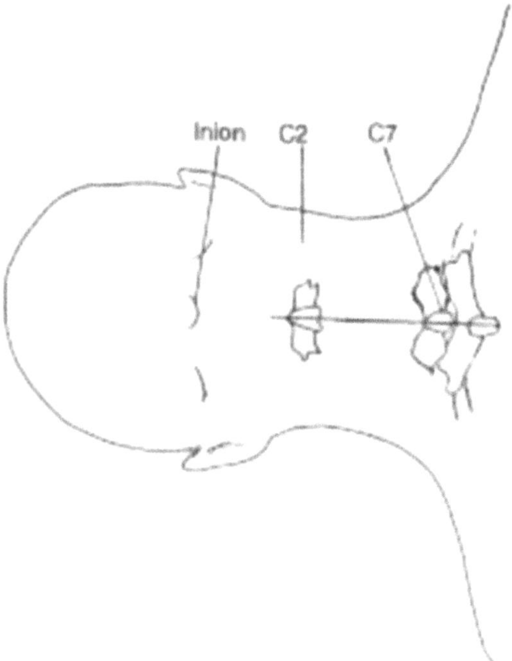

Fig. 3. Guides to a midline incision

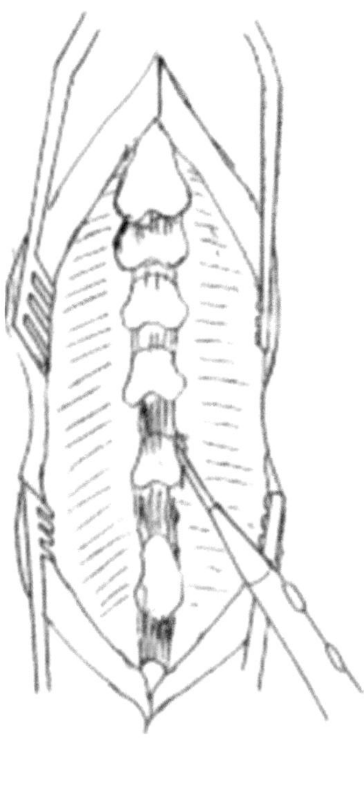

Fig. 4. Exposure of the tips of the spinous processes after division of the nuchal ligament

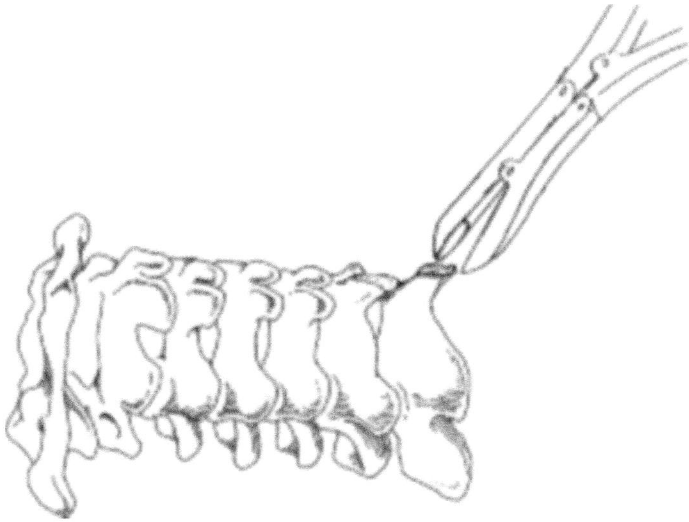

Fig. 5. Partial resection of the C6 and C7 spinous processes to match their length with those of C3, C4, and C5

Open Side Gutter Formation and Flavectomy

Once the paracervical muscles are detached from the laminae, retractors are put in place to hold the surgical field, and the open side gutter is made first at the junction of the laminae and the facet joints with a steel bur (Fig. 6a,b). The ventral cortex can either be resected with a thin-bladed Kerrison rongeur, or perforated with a diamond bur (Fig. 6c). We prefer the latter to avoid excessive bleeding from the epidural venous plexus. When bleeding from the epidural venous plexus is encountered, it can be managed effectively by a gentle pack of hemostatic agents such as Novacol (Bioplex, Montdale, NJ, USA) or Avitene (Davol, Woburn, MA, USA).

The ligamentum flavum at the upper and lower ends of the laminar door, usually at C2/3 and C7/T1, are resected with a thin-bladed Kerrison rongeur while opening the interspace with a small lamina spreader (Fig. 7).

Hinge Side Gutter Formation and Placement of Stay Sutures

The bony gutter on the hinge side then is made with a high-speed bur slightly more lateral than the one on the open side. While drilling, the stability of the hinge is checked frequently by applying a gentle bending force to the spinous processes to prevent hinge breakage (Fig. 8). When all the spinous processes and laminae become slightly mobile yet retain a spring-like resistance, the laminar door is ready to be opened. At this point, pieces of suture are placed through the zygoapophyseal articular capsules and the surrounding soft tissue at each level in the hinge side and are passed through

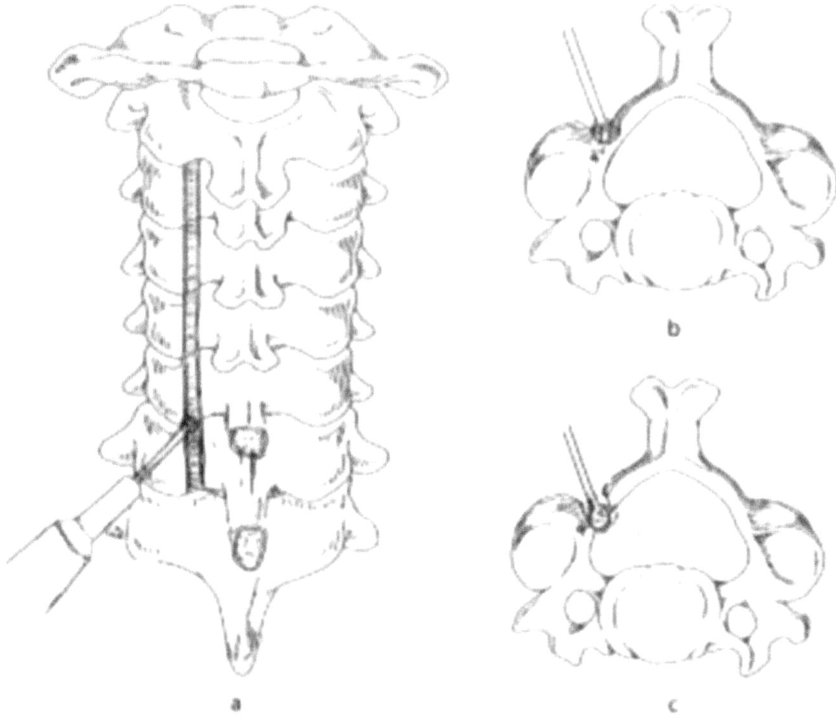

Fig. 6. Formation of the open side gutter. **a, b**, Drilling with a steel bur; **c** perforation of the ventral cortex with a diamond bur

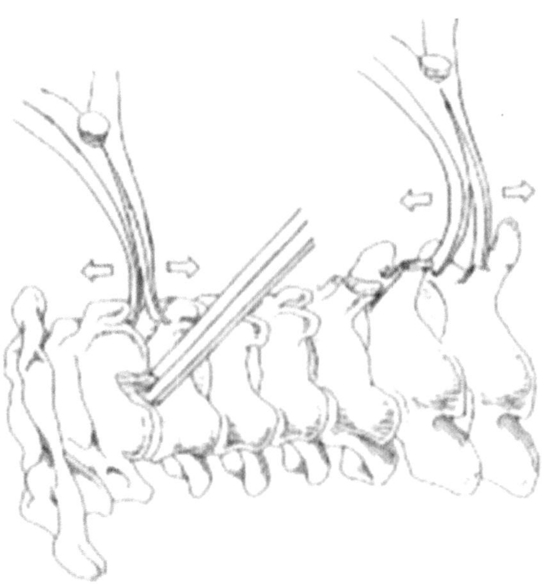

Fig. 7. Removal of the ligamentum flavum with a fine-tipped Kerrison rongeur while opening the interspace with a custom-made lamina spreader

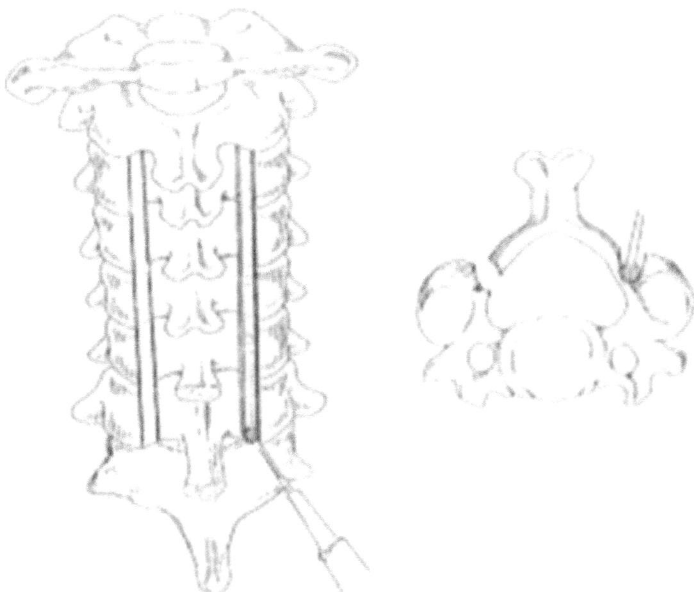

Fig. 8. Formation of the hinge side gutter. A wider gutter is made at a slightly more lateral position than the one on the open side

interspinous ligaments around the base of the corresponding spinous process because this cannot be done once the laminae are opened (Fig. 9).

Canal Expansion

Just prior to opening the laminar door, the patient's neck position is changed from a flexed to a neutral position. The tip of the blade of a large Kerrison rongeur is placed under the excised margin of one of the laminae in the open side and the edge is lifted slightly (Fig. 10). The spinous process is held in the expanded position by the fingers of an assistant. Then the next lamina is lifted in the same manner until all the laminae have been opened to the same extent. This procedure is repeated slowly and the laminar door is opened gradually. In the middle of the opening process, the remaining fibrous tissues in the open side, including the ligamentum flavum, should be excised with scissors or a spatula because they become tense and prevent laminar opening. Adhesions between the laminae and the dura should also be released with the spatula. Significant bleeding from the epidural venous plexus is usually encountered at this point, but can be managed with bipolar coagulation and/or a gentle pack with hemostatic materials. Do not try to open one lamina completely in one attempt or the hinge will break. Usually, dural pulsation can be observed in the middle of the opening procedure

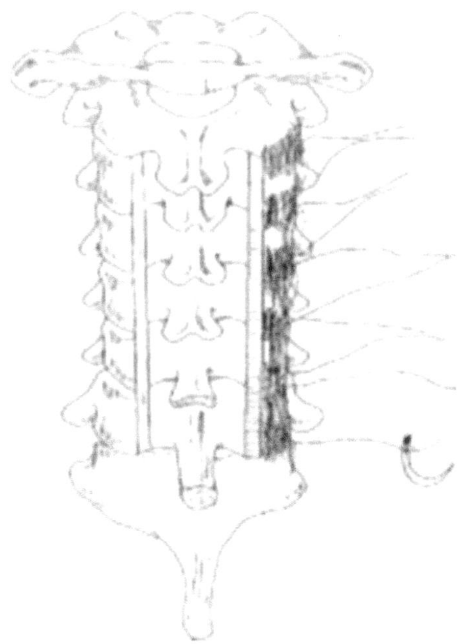

Fig. 9. Stay sutures are passed through the facet joint capsules and adjacent soft tissue just before the opening procedure

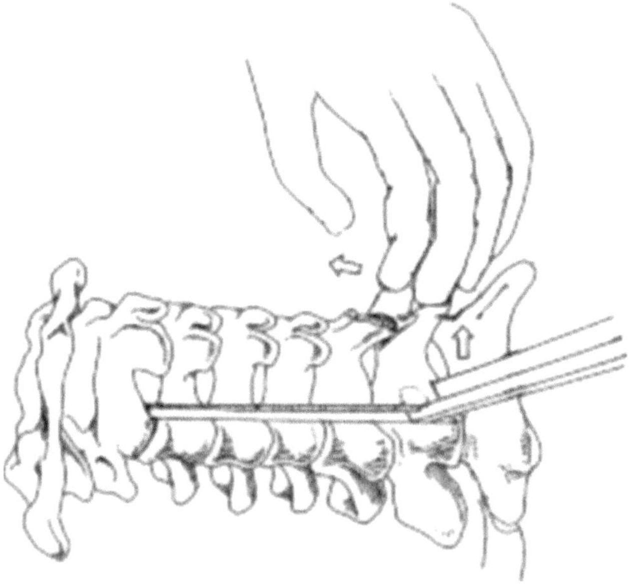

Fig. 10. Opening procedure. The tip of a large Kerrison rongeur is placed underneath the excised lamina in the open side and lifted slightly. The lifted position is held by the fingers of an assistant. This procedure is repeated for all the laminae until they are all open to the same extent. Then the whole process is repeated until the laminar door is completely opened

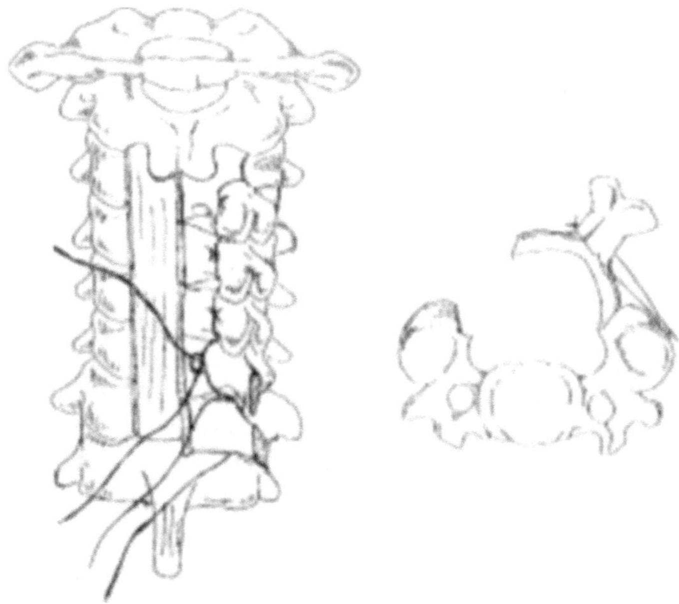

Fig. 11. The stay sutures are passed around the base of the spinous processes and tied tightly to hold the laminae in the opened position

before complete expansion. These maneuvers should be continued until the laminae of the open side become almost horizontal.

Stay Sutures

To maintain the expanded position and to prevent reclosure, threads previously placed at the base of the spinous processes are securely tied (Fig. 11). More than sufficient space for decompression can be obtained between the swollen dural tube and the lamina. It is important to open the laminar door as much as possible, especially in cases of OPLL, because the laminae are pushed back slightly while closing the muscle layers.

Wound Closure

A drainage tube is placed in the epidural space. Bilateral neck muscles are approximated to minimize the dead space and the nuchal ligaments are tightly sutured with nonabsorbable sutures.

Postoperative Care

Postoperatively, the patient is allowed to walk at 3 days with a soft collar, which is worn until the patient becomes sufficiently confident to remove the brace, usually after about a week. After removal of the collar, the patient is encouraged to start gentle range-of-motion (ROM) exercises of the neck. The stitches are removed 10 days postoperatively. The patient is encouraged to return to work after 3–4 weeks. Rigorous activities, including sports, are usually permitted 3 months postoperatively.

Surgical Results

Neurological Recovery

The surgical results of 80 patients who underwent ELAP for cervical spondylotic myelopathy (CSM) or OPLL with at least 10 years follow-up were reviewed (Fig. 12) [24, 25]. There were 27 patients with CSM (23 men and 4 women, average age at the time of surgery 51.6 years) and 53 with OPLL (42 men and 11 women, average age at the time of surgery 56.0 years). The follow-up period averaged 14.1 years for CSM patients and 14.3 years for OPLL patients. In CSM patients, the mean Japanese Orthopaedic Association (JOA) score of 8.4 preoperatively improved to 13.8 (average recovery rate 57.9%) at 3 years and was maintained at 13.1 (55.7%) at the final follow-

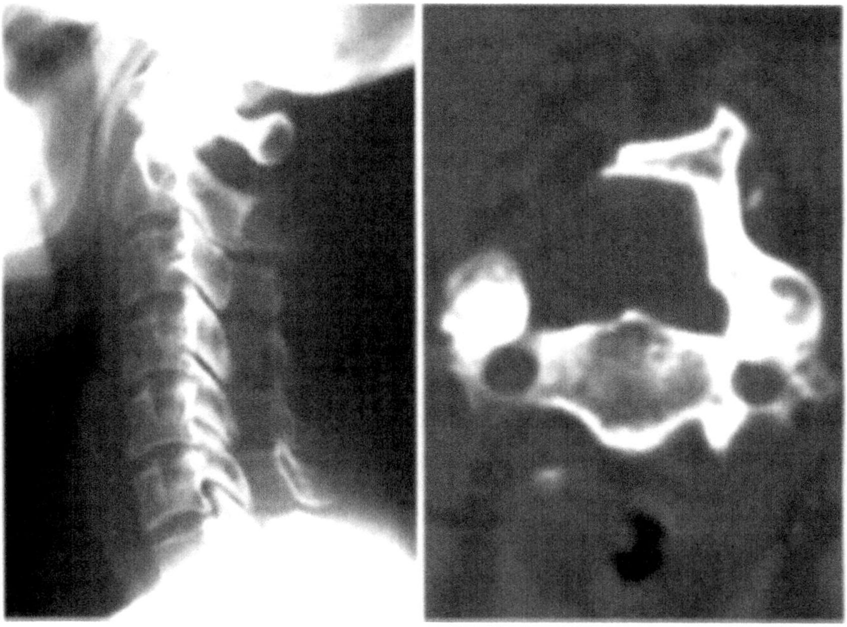

Fig. 12. Expansive laminoplasty in a 56-year-old female patient with cervical spondylosis. **a** Sufficient expansion of the anteroposterior diameter of the spinal canal between C3 and C7 is evident on a lateral radiograph. **b** A computed tomography scan reveals sufficient expansion of the cross-sectional area of the spinal canal with bony fusion of the hinge

up. The mean JOA score (8.3 preoperatively) and recovery rate of OPLL patients also reached the maximum at 3 years postoperatively (13.8 and 63.3%, respectively), and were maintained at satisfactory levels at the final follow-up (12.7 and 47.9%, respectively). Overall, 59.3% of the patients were rated as either excellent or good for CSM, and 55.0% for OPLL. Late gradual neurological deterioration, mainly in lower extremity motor function, developed in 7 CSM patients and 16 OPLL patients whose mean age at the final follow-up were 70 and 77 years, respectively. The probable causes of the deterioration included comorbidities such as cerebrovascular, heart, and degenerative lumbar diseases, as well as a progression of OPLL. However, such motor dysfunction may partly be due to normal aging processes. A correction for age may be necessary for an appropriate assessment of the actual effect of surgery on neurological functions, particularly in elderly patients, in long-term follow-up studies.

Surgical Stresses

The operating time averaged 2h 8min for CSM and 2h 10min for OPLL, and the average amount of bleeding was 393g for CSM and 493g for OPLL patients.

Axial Symptoms

Complaints about shoulder stiffness and axial pain at the final follow-up were received from 33% and 28%, respectively, of the total number of patients in the CSM groups and from 41% and 25%, respectively, of the total number of patients in the OPLL group. However, fewer than 10% of the patients in both groups were taking daily antiinflammatory drugs because of such symptoms.

Radiographical Findings

Degree of Expansion

The average AP diameter at the C4 level on plain lateral radiograms in patients with CSM was 11.5mm preoperatively. That increased to 18.2mm at 1 year postoperatively and was maintained at 17.4mm at the final follow-up. One patient had a recurrence of myelopathy due to reclosure of the opened laminae.

The preoperative AP diameter at C4 in OPLL patients averaged 13.5mm. That increased to 18.3mm at 1 year postoperatively and was maintained at 17.9mm at the final follow-up. However, a decrease in the space available for the cord (SAC) associated with a postoperative progression of ossification was observed in over 60% of the patients.

Progression of OPLL

A progression of ossification was found in 66% of patients with OPLL, and the percentage of patients with continuous-type OPLL increased from 26% to 53%. However, although patients with such progression had lower recovery rates, no statistically significant difference in the final JOA scores was detected between those with and without progression. This, along with the findings in a different study [5] in which the postoperative progression of continuous and mixed types of OPLL was 89% in the laminectomy group, 34% in the laminoplasty group, and 20% in the anterior spinal fusion group, indicating an inability of ELAP to prevent progression of OPLL, may support our contention that a wider and longer decompression may be necessary for patients with OPLL.

Sufficient decompression was verified in postoperative MR images in both CSM and OPLL patients, although asymptomatic, degenerative changes at the cranial and caudal ends of the laminar expansion were found in 57% of the patients who underwent MRI examination and need further observation.

Alignment

In the CSM group, the percentage of patients with lordosis decreased from 70% preoperatively to 52% at the final follow-up, and patients with nonlordotic alignment increased accordingly. The same trend was found in the OPLL group, in which the percentage decreased from 69% preoperatively to 51% at the final follow-up. Severe kyphotic deformity did not develop in any patient in either group. Even though there were no significant differences in the final recovery rates among patients with different alignments in the CSM and OPLL groups, patients with kyphosis in the OPLL group had a much lower mean recovery rate (9%) than those with lordosis (52%) or with a straight spine (38%).

Range of Motion

Postoperative ROM between C2 and C7 decreased significantly from 44° to 14° at the final follow-up in the CSM group, and from 32° to 11° in the OPLL group, while that between the occiput and C2 increased slightly from 22° to 28° in the CSM group and from 23° to 25° in the OPLL group, giving a mean overall decrease of 37% in CSM patients and 35% in OPLL patients on flexion extension radiographs.

Twenty-seven percent of CSM patients and 38% of OPLL patients had complaints about a restricted ROM. These were mainly difficulties in turning their head to look their shoulder or in looking down at the tips of their toes, and most of them had minor disturbances in the activities of daily living (ADL).

A decrease in ROM due to fusion at the hinge side may stabilize the spine and maintain favorable long-term results, while at the same time it may become a source of axial complaints. However, this downside is to some extent compensated for by preserved upper cervical spine motion resulting in less ADL disturbance.

Complications

The motor weakness in the C5 or C6 segments that developed in two CSM patients and six OPLL patients was the most serious complication, although most of these recovered completely within 2 years postoperatively. The details of the complications, including segmental motor palsy, are discussed elsewhere in this volume (see chapters by Matsumoto and Chiba).

Cautions and Tips

Since the advent of ELAP in 1977, a number of revisions have been made and options have been added to the original technique [5, 12, 22]. The retention sutures placed around the base of the spinous processes, securing the lamina to the corresponding joint capsules, is one of them. This was introduced from our early experiences in which reoperation was necessary because of reclosure of the laminae [18].

We currently use a disposable anchor screw system (PeBA Anchor Screw, Smith and Nephew, Orthopaedic Biosystem, Andover, MA, USA) to hold the lamina more securely and accurately in position. These screws can be placed in the lateral mass, and solid bony purchases can be obtained (Fig. 13).

In our early cases, in which both gutters were made simultaneously, we occasionally experienced breakage of the hinge, which may lead to serious neurological demise, while excising the ventral cortex of the open side with a Kerrison rongeur. We therefore changed the sequence of the procedures so that the hinge gutter is made after the completion of all other procedures, including the resection of the ventral cortex in the open side and the ligamentum flavum, to avoid such breakage [12, 22].

The postoperative curvature plays a vital role in the decompression mechanism of ELAP by allowing a dorsal shift of the spinal cord, especially in OPLL cases in which patients with postoperative kyphosis tend to deteriorate [7, 22, 26–28]. On the other hand, the difference in the cervical alignment did not affect the surgical results in patients with CSM. In patients with CSM, the redundancy induced in the spinal cord through multiple disc degeneration may dissipate the compression on the spinal cord even in the kyphotic alignment, while patients with OPLL are less likely to have such a

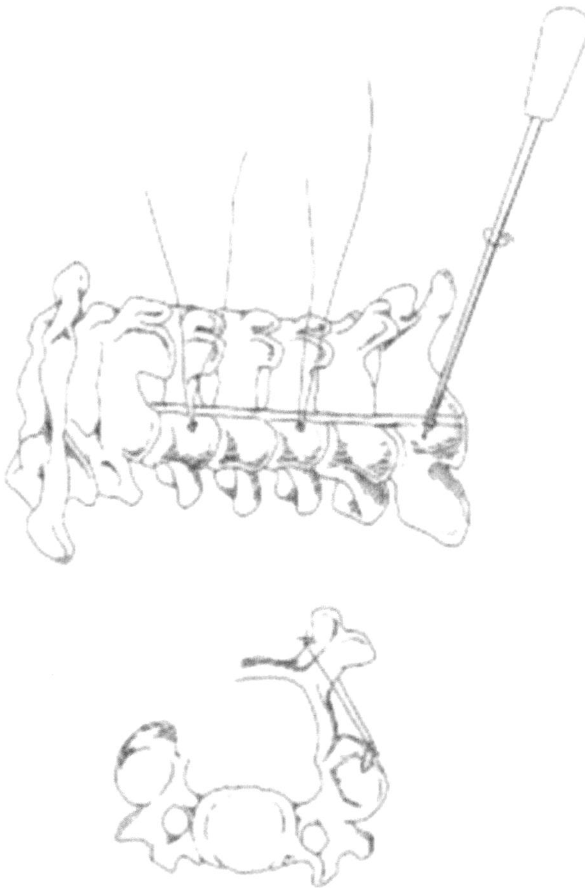

Fig. 13. The use of the PeBA Anchoring Screw System as stay sutures

redundancy in the spinal cord because the ossified ligament holds the vertical height of the cervical spine and maintains compression on the spinal cord [29].

To maintain and reinforce cervical lordosis, the spinous process of C2 should be excluded from the laminar expansion to preserve the attachment of the semispinalis muscles whenever possible. Just before the laminar opening, the patient's neck position is changed from a flexed to a neutral position to maintain and secure cervical lordosis. This allows the surgeon to confirm the lordotic alignment directly in the operative field, and stay sutures can be tied and the reconstruction of the muscular layers can be done in the neutral position [5, 12, 22].

We also preserve the supraspinous and interspinous ligaments as much as possible to maintain cervical lordosis. In some cases, these ligaments at the caudal end of the laminar door become tight and exert strong resistance when opening the laminae, making sufficient expansion difficult. In such cases, the spinous process just below the caudal end of the expansion, usually that of T1, is exposed, and an osteotomy is carried out with a high-speed drill at the base of the spinous process, which is bent toward the hinge side to relieve the tension of these ligaments [5, 22].

Secure neck muscle reconstruction followed by early active exercise is also important to preserve the cervical lordosis. However, even though the preservation of the preoperative alignment has been possible to a certain degree, to date, no one has succeeded in reversing the preoperatively established kyphosis into physiological lordosis [5].

Various modifications have been developed that use bone grafts or spacers to try to address problems of reclosure or cervical alignment, but we feel that no spacers or grafts are necessary if the cautions mentioned above are followed.

In patients with OPLL, it is also recommended that the spinal canal be expanded more extensively in both the sagittal and transverse planes, because a progression of OPLL in either a longitudinal or a transverse direction was present in 66% of patients. This may be caused by biological stimulation attributable to surgical invasion, biomechanical stresses, or hereditary disposition. In our previous series, in which all patients underwent expansion of the same extent the recovery rates of those with a significant increase in OPLL were lower than in those without an increase. We therefore expand the laminae as much as possible in the axial plane, and as far as one level below and above the site of compression in the sagittal plane. We have included C2 in the levels of decompression in 60% of the patients and obtained favorable results [22, 25].

References

1. Kirita Y (1976) Posterior decompression for cervical spondylosis and OPLL. (in Japanese) Shujutsu 30:287–302
2. Cattell HS, Clark GL (1967) Cervical kyphosis and instability following multiple laminectomies in children. J Bone Joint Surg 49A:713–721
3. Kawai S, Sunago K, Doi K, et al. (1988) Cervical laminoplasty (Hattori's method). Procedure and follow-up results. Spine 13:1245–1250
4. Ohyama M, Hattori S, Moriwaki N, et al. (1973) A new method of cervical laminectomy. (in Japanese) Chubu Nippon Siekeigeka Gakkai Zasshi 16:792–794
5. Hirabayashi K, Toyama Y, Chiba K (1999) Expansive laminoplasty for myelopathy in ossification of the longitudinal ligament. Clin Orthop 1359:35–48

6. Hirabayashi K (1978) Expansive open-door laminoplasty for cervical spondylotic myelopathy. (in Japanese) Shujutsu 32:1159–1163
7. Fujimura Y, Nishi Y, Nakamura M (1997) Dorsal shift and expansion of the spinal cord after expansive open-door laminoplasty. J Spinal Disord 10:282–287
8. Herkowitz HN (1988) Cervical laminaplasty: its role in the treatment of cervical radiculopathy. J Spinal Disord 1:179–188
9. Norwinski GP, Visarius H, Nolte LP, et al. (1993) A biomechanical comparison of cervical laminaplasty and cervical laminectomy with progressive facetectomy. Spine 18:1995–2004
10. Yonenobu K, Hosono N, Iwasaki M, et al. (1992) Laminoplasty versus subtotal corpectomy. A comparative study of results in multisegmental cervical spondylotic myelopathy. Spine 17:1281–1284
11. Baba H, Furusawa N, Imura S, et al. (1994) Laminoplasty following anterior cervical fusion for spondylotic myeloradiculopathy. Int Orthop 18:1–5
12. Hirabayashi K (1994) Expansive open-door laminoplasty. In: Sherk HH, Dunn EJ, Eismont FJ (eds) The cervical spine. An atlas of surgical procedures. Lippincott, Philadelphia, pp 233–250
13. Herkowitz HN (1988) A comparison of anterior cervical fusion, cervical laminectomy, and cervical laminoplasty for the surgical management of multiple level spondylotic radiculopathy. Spine 13:774–780
14. Satomi K, Nishi Y, Kohno T, et al. (1994) Long-term follow-up studies of open-door expansive laminoplasty for cervical stenotic myelopathy. Spine 19:507–510
15. Iwasaki M, Ebara S, Miyamoto S, et al. (1996) Expansive laminoplasty for cervical radiculomyelopathy due to soft disc herniation. Spine 21:32–38
16. Yonenobu K, Fuji T, Ono K, et al. (1985) Choice of surgical treatment for multisegmental cervical spondylotic myelopathy. Spine 10:710–716
17. Shinomiya K, Okamoto A, Kamikozuru M, et al. (1993) An analysis of failures in primary cervical anterior spinal cord decompression and fusion. J Spinal Disord 6: 277–288
18. Hirabayashi K, Watanabe K, Wakano K, et al. (1983) Expansive open-door laminoplasty for cervical spinal stenotic myelopathy. Spine 8:693–699
19. Toyama Y, Hirabayashi H, Kamata M, et al. (1997) Long-term clinical results of anterior interbody fusion for cervical spondylotic myelopathy. (in Japanese) J East Jpn Orthop Traumatol 9:487–492
20. Hirabayashi K, Toyama Y (1997) Choice of surgical procedure for cervical ossification of the posterior longitudinal ligaments. In: Yonenobu K, Sakou T, Ono K (eds) Ossification of the posterior longitudinal ligament. Springer, Tokyo, pp 135–142
21. Fujimura Y, Nishi Y, Chiba K, et al. (1998) Multiple regression analysis of the factors influencing the results of expansive open-door laminoplasty for cervical myelopathy due to ossification of the posterior longitudinal ligament. Arch Orthop Trauma Surg 117:471–474
22. Hirabayashi K, Satomi K, Toyama Y (1998) Surgical management of OPLL: anterior versus posterior approach. Part II. In: The Cervical Spine Research Society Editorial Committee (eds) The cervical spine, 3rd edn. Lippincott-Raven, Philadelphia, pp 876–887
23. Baba H, Maezawa Y, Furusawa N, et al. (1995) Flexibility and alignment of the cervical spine after laminoplasty for spondylotic myelopathy. A radiographic study. Int Orthop 19:116–121

24. Maruiwa H, Chiba K, Watanabe M, et al. (2000) Long-term results of expansive open-door laminoplasty for cervical spondylotic myelopathy. (in Japanese) Rinsho Seikeigeka 35:411–416
25. Maruiwa H, Kamata M, Watanabe M, et al. (2000) Long-term results of expansive open-door laminoplasty for ossification of the longitudinal ligament. (in Japanese) J Jpn Orthop Assoc 74:S690
26. Baba H, Uchida K, Maezawa Y, et al. (1996) Lordotic alignment and posterior migration of the spinal cord following en bloc open-door laminoplasty for cervical myelopathy: a magnetic resonance imaging study. J Neurol 243:626–632
27. Kimura I, Shingu H, Nasu Y (1995) Long-term follow-up of cervical spondylotic myelopathy treated by canal-expansive laminoplasty. J Bone Joint Surg Br 77:956–961
28. Kohno K, Kumon Y, Oka Y, et al. (1997) Evaluation of prognostic factors following expansive laminoplasty for cervical spinal stenotic myelopathy. Surg Neurol 48: 237–245
29. Chiba K, Toyama Y, Watanabe M, et al. (2000) Impact of longitudinal distance of the cervical spine on the results of expansive open-door laminoplasty. Spine 25: 2893–2898

Double-Door Laminoplasty by Splitting Spinous Processes

Atsushi Seichi, Motoshige Iwasaki, and Kozo Nakamura

The Concept of Double-Door Laminoplasty

Until the 1970s, laminectomy had been the sole therapeutic option for posterior decompression of the spinal cord. However, wide laminectomy of the cervical spine sometimes caused early and/or late neurological deterioration. The possible causes of such deterioration were the progression of malalignments such as kyphosis or listhesis, postoperative progression of ossification of the posterior longitudinal ligament (OPLL) associated with malalignment and instability of the cervical spine in cases with OPLL, and massive scar formation in the epidural space, known as "postlaminectomy membrane" [1–4]. To resolve the problems associated with laminectomy, several variations of laminoplasty have been developed in Japan [5–7]. Double-door laminoplasty was developed by Kurokawa et al., and a preliminary report was published in 1982 [8]. The main aim of this laminoplasty was to expand the spinal canal symmetrically while preserving the mobility of the cervical spine. In common with other kinds of laminoplasty, the aims of this procedure to preserve the posterior structure in the midline of the cervical spine were to prevent postoperative progression of malalignment and instability of the cervical spine, and to protect the spinal cord from postlaminectomy membrane. In addition, one potential advantage of this procedure was that it preserved the long spinous processes as posterior stabilizers of the neck [8]. Compared with Hattori's Z-laminoplasty, double-door laminoplasty is technically straightforward. Compared with unilateral hinge-type laminoplasty, such as Hirabayashi's method, double-door laminoplasty has some theoretical and practical advantages: symmetrical expansion of the spinal canal, avoidance of hemorrhage from the epidural veins because of the limited number of these veins in the midline, and the potential for posterior fusion with a bone graft bridge between the spinous processes.

Department of Orthopaedic Surgery, Faculty of Medicine, The University of Tokyo, 7-3-1 Hongo, Bunkyo-ku, Tokyo 113-0033, Japan

Indications

Cervical myelopathy, caused by multisegmental stenotic conditions due to spondylosis or OPLL, is an indication for double-door laminoplasty. This method is also indicated for localized anterior cord compression due to disc herniation, spondylosis, or OPLL level when these pathologies are complicated by congenital or developmental spinal canal stenosis. Since the mechanism is posterior decompression of the spinal cord, the kyphotic cervical spine is theoretically not a good indication. However, when the kyphosis is mild, positive surgical effects can be expected [9]. The surgical effects for patients with severely kyphotic cervical spine remain unknown. Double-door laminoplasty has also been applied to patients with cervical stenotic myelopathy due to rheumatoid arthritis and athetoid cerebral palsy. Cord tumors can be resected through the posterior approach when they are located in the posterior side.

Invasiveness of laminoplasty

In the original procedure by Kurokawa, small bone blocks from the iliac crest were grafted to the split spinous processes [8, 9]. Using this method, the average operative time was about 5 h, and average intraoperative bleeding was about 700 g. Recently, in order to decrease the operation time and blood loss and to avoid postoperative pain around the donor site of the graft, an artificial spacer often has been used as an alternative to an autograft in other hospitals as well as ours [10] (see the chapter by S. Harata in this volume). The use of an artificial spacer has shortened the average operative time and reduced intraoperative bleeding. In 1999, 26 patients had double-door laminoplasty with hydroxyapatite spacers at Tokyo University Hospital; patients who had surgery to the thoracic or lumbar spine during the same operation were excluded. The average operation time was 216 min (105–300 min), the average intraoperative blood loss was 247 g (60–990 g), and no transfusions were necessary. The operative time and intraoperative bleeding are, of course, governed by the surgeon's learning curve. To perform laminoplasty safely, competent handling of the air-drill is essential, but for a trained spinal surgeon, double-door laminoplasty is now a safe procedure. Since the epidural venous plexuses run mainly over the posterolateral aspect of the cord, rather than the midline, bleeding while opening the midline is easily managed using a bipolar coagulator and gel forms soaked in thrombin.

Procedure

The area of the laminoplasty is determined by preoperative magnetic resonance imaging (MRI). Laminoplasty between C3 and C7 is common, and C2 is sometimes included. The patient is placed on a modified Hall frame in the prone position. Intraoperative blood pressure should be maintained at around 100 mmHg by the anesthesiologist to ensure easy control of intraoperative bleeding. A midline skin incision is employed. A posterior approach is made along the edge of the nuchal ligament to the line of the spinous processes (Fig. 1a). Using this approach, the continuity of the nuchal ligament can be maintained. The semispinalis cervicis is then transiently detached from the C2 spinous process (Fig. 1b) [11]. In a case where the surgical field extends to C1 and C2, detachment of the rectus capitis posterior major and obliqus capitis inferior muscles is carried out (Fig. 1c). The cervical laminae are exposed laterally to the center of the facet joint, and interspinous ligaments and muscles are removed using a rongeur. The spinous processes are sagitally split to the base with a 2-mm-diameter steel burr, and the separation is completed with a 2-mm-diameter diamond burr. After bilateral troughs (grooves) for the hinges are carefully made with a 3–4-mm-diameter diamond burr at the transitional area between the facet joint and laminae (Fig. 2), spinal canal enlargement is achieved by opening the split laminae bilaterally with a specially designed laminae spreader (TACT Medical, Tokyo, Japan, Fig. 3). Preoperative computed tomography (CT) is helpful to determine the exact position of the lateral troughs. The surgeon should confirm that the hinges preserve their elasticity and that the opening of the split laminae is symmetrical.

Using the laminae spreader, the surgeon can measure the size of the spacer to be inserted (Fig. 4). Spinal canal enlargement is maintained by placing appropriately sized coricocancellous bone blocks obtained from the iliac crest, or artificial spacers, which are held in place with sutures passed through holes made in the spinous processes (Fig. 5). C3–C7 is a typical area of laminoplasty (Fig. 6). The dome-like osteotomy of C2 is added if necessary (Fig. 7). To decompress the cord up to C1, the posterior arch of C1 is resected (Fig. 8). When posterior spinal fusion is required, one long iliac bone block is placed between the spinous processes to be fused and secured with sutures or wires (Fig. 9). If posterolateral fusion is required, bone tips are placed over the troughs.

Before closing the wound, the surgeon should confirm that the dural tube is well decompressed, and is not constricted between the split spinous processes. The use of a free fat graft over the dural tube is controversial. The detached muscles are then reattached to the spinous process of C2 (Fig. 10). Preservation of the continuity of the nuchal ligament and reconstruction of the erector spinae muscles to the C2 are important in order to maintain

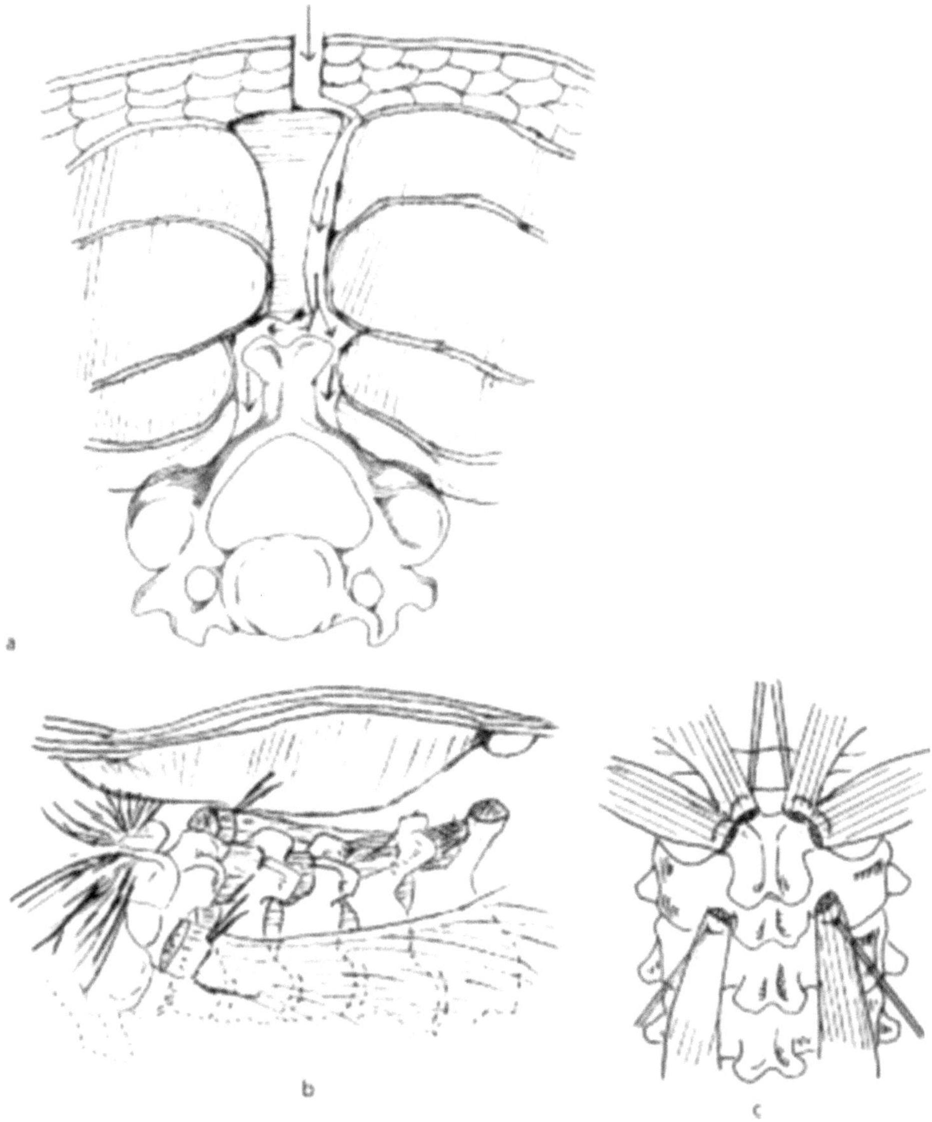

Fig. 1. **a** The *arrows* show the posterior approach to the cervical laminae. The approach is made along the edge of the nuchal ligament. The most superficial muscle, the trapezius, is separated from the superior nuchal ligament and the spinous process of C7. The splenius capitis muscles are also detached from the nuchal ligament. This approach preserves the continuity of the nuchal ligament. **b** The nuchal ligament is preserved. The semispinalis cervicis is transiently detached from the C2 spinous process to allow access from C3 to C7. **c** When C1 and C2 are included in the decompressive area, rectus capitis posterior major and obliquus capitis inferior muscles are detached

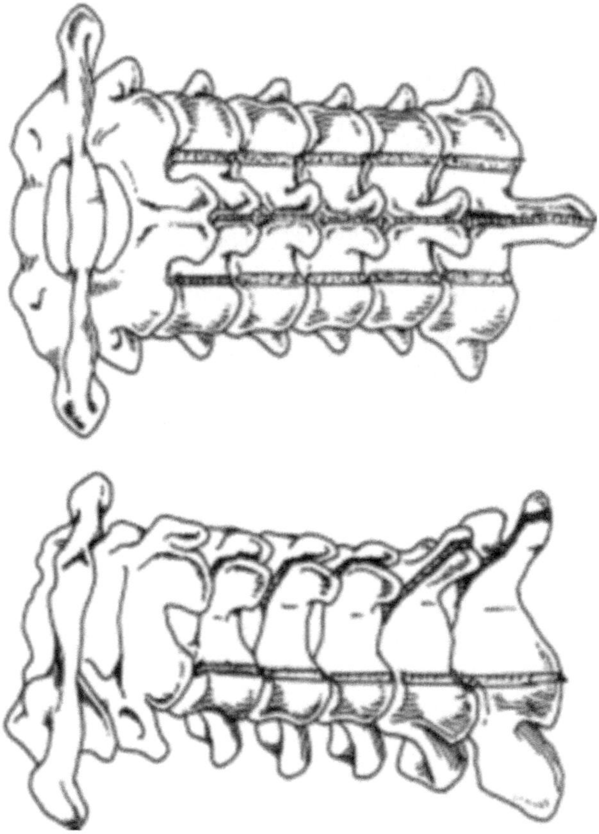

Fig. 2. Spinous processes are sagitally split and bilateral troughs (bony grooves) for the hinges are made at the transitional area between the facet joint and the laminae

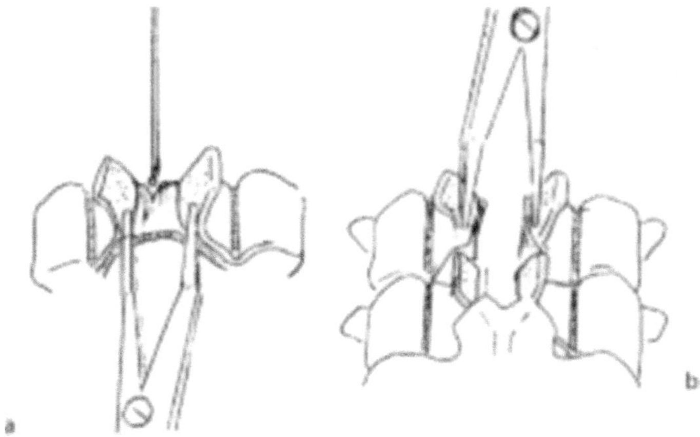

Fig. 3. The split spinous process and lamina is opened using a lamina spreader. The ligamentum flavum is split with a microprobe. The lamina spreader shows the appropriate size of the spacers to be inserted in the split spinous process

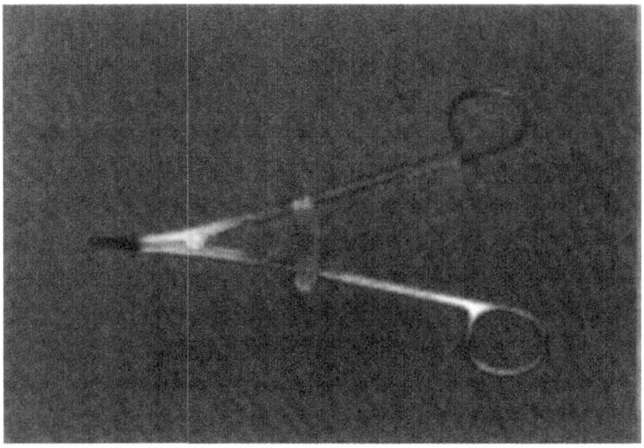

Fig. 4. The lamina spreader is helpful to open the split spinous process and determine the size of the spacer needed

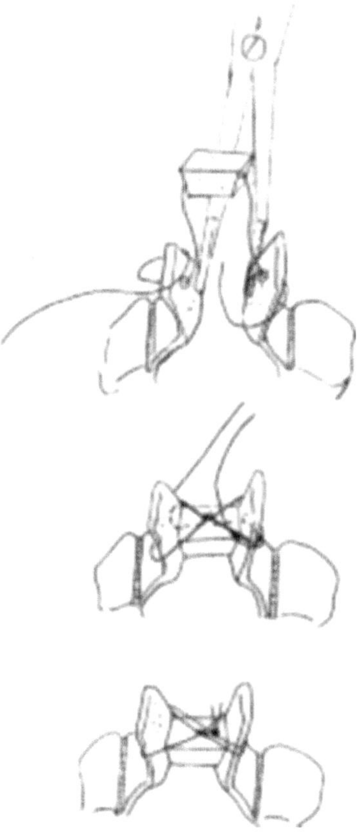

Fig. 5. A hydroxyapatite spacer or iliac bone block is held in place with sutures passing through holes made in the spinous process

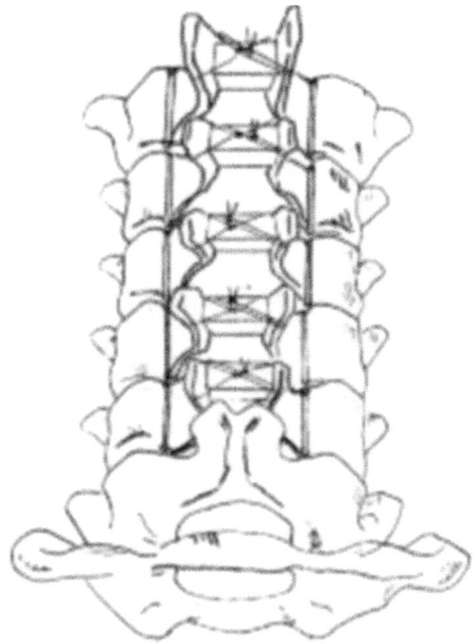

Fig. 6. Laminoplasty from C3 to C7 is completed

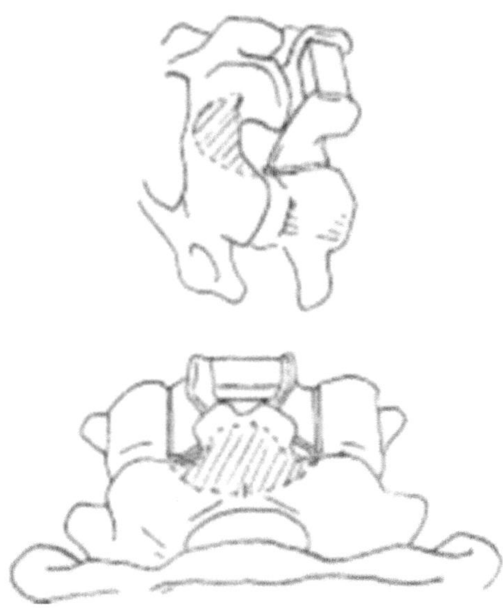

Fig. 7. To extend the decompressive area toward C2, dome-like laminoplasty for C2 can be performed without detaching the rectus capitis posterior or obliqus capitis inferior muscles

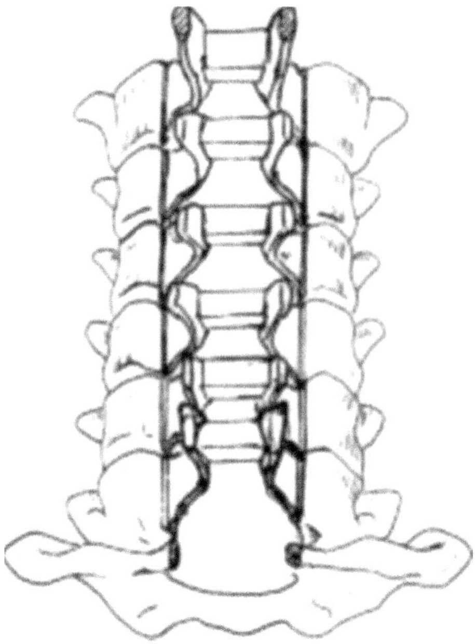

Fig. 8. Laminectomy of C1 and laminoplasty from C2 to C7

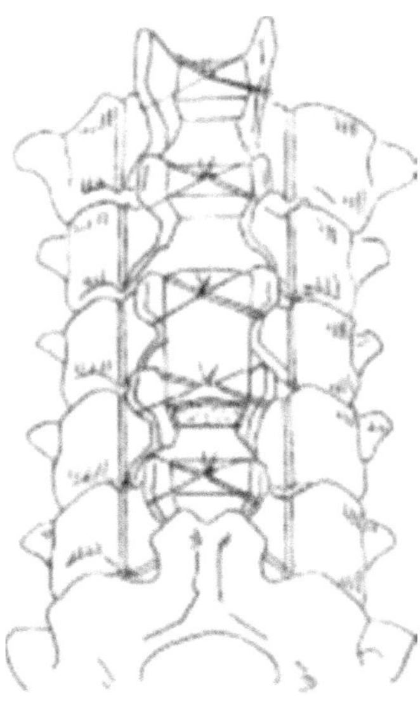

Fig. 9. Posterior spinal fusion is accomplished by placing one long iliac bone block between the spinous processes to be fused

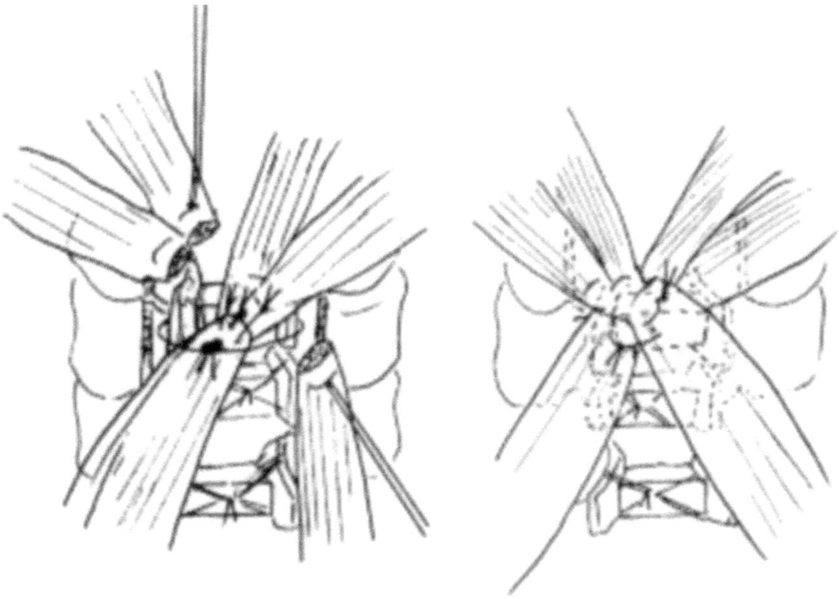

Fig. 10. Reconstruction of the deep muscles detached from C2

cervical extensor power and cervical alignment. A suction drainage tube is set over the laminae. The trapezius muscle is tightly sutured with the nuchal ligament. Finally, the superficial layers and skin are sutured individually.

Technical Points

To split spinous processes safely, a cranial part of the base of the spinous processes is fenestrated. By this procedure, the surgeon can split the spinous processes under direct visualization (Fig. 11). Lateral troughs should not be made too medial or too lateral. Troughs which are too medial make for insufficient enlargement of the spinal canal, which causes constriction of the dural tube between the split spinous processes. On the other hand, troughs which are too lateral make opening the split laminae difficult. Preoperative planning using CT helps the surgeon to make appropriate troughs. Care should be taken not to make the troughs too deep, which makes the laminae unstable. Each lamina should be opened gently, little by little, to achieve simultaneous decompression of the entire cervical cord. To open one lamina rapidly in isolation may cause the hinges to break, or may disturb simultaneous decompression of the entire cervical cord. If a lamina becomes unstable owing to a trough which is too deep, this lamina should be resected. Thin spinous processes are difficult to split. Oblique osteotomy is recom-

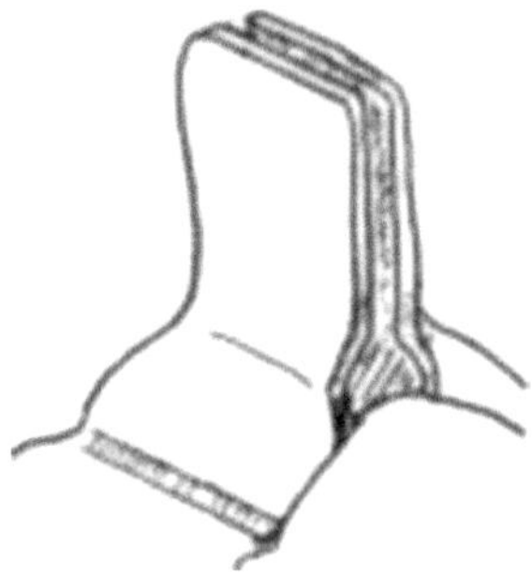

Fig. 11. Fenestration of a cranial part of the base of the spinous processes makes it possible for surgeons to split the spinous processes under direct visualization

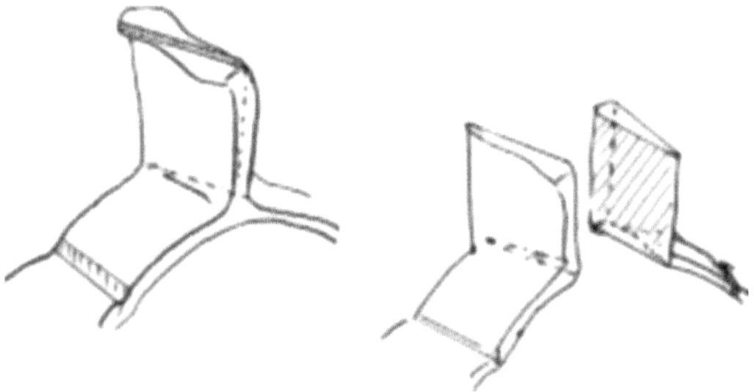

Fig. 12. Thin spinous processes can be split by oblique osteotomy

mended when splitting a thin spinous process (Fig. 12). If a spinous process is broken during midline osteotomy, the Nara Medical College method (see the chapter by H. Iwasaki in this volume) or laminectomy of the broken site are options.

Postoperative Management

The patient is allowed and encouraged to stand up and walk after removal of the suction drain, within a week after the operation. A simple cervical collar is used postoperatively for 3 weeks.

Results

Long-Term Results (Over 10 Years) of Double-Door Laminoplasty Using Autogenous Iliac Bone Grafts

Sixty patients with cervical stenotic myelopathy underwent double-door laminoplasty using an autogenous iliac bone graft between 1980 and 1988, and were followed for the next 10 years. There were 43 men and 17 women, and the average age at surgery was 55 years (range 36–69 years). The average follow-up period was 154 months (range 120–218 months). Of the 60 patients, 35 had cervical myelopathy caused by ossification of the OPLL in the cervical spine, and 25 had cervical spondylotic myelopathy, including 5 with athetoid cerebral palsy. The severity of their clinical symptoms was assessed using an evaluation score established by the Japanese Orthopaedic Association (JOA score). The results of surgery were estimated by Kurokawa's method, based on the scores of motor dysfunction of the upper and lower extremities (Table 1) [8, 9].

In 33 of the 35 patients with OPLL (92%), the surgical results by Kurokawa's method were fair or better 1 year after surgery (Fig. 13). In 25

Table 1. Grade of surgical results estimated by Kurokawa's method based on the scores of motor dysfunction in the upper and lower extremities [8]

Excellent. The scores of both upper and lower extremities improved ≧1, and those of either extremity improved ≧2
Good. The score of either of both extremities improved ≧1, and neither became worse
Fair. The function of one extremity improved without a rise in score, and neither became worse
Unchanged. No change in function of either extremity
Poor. The function of either or both extremities became worse

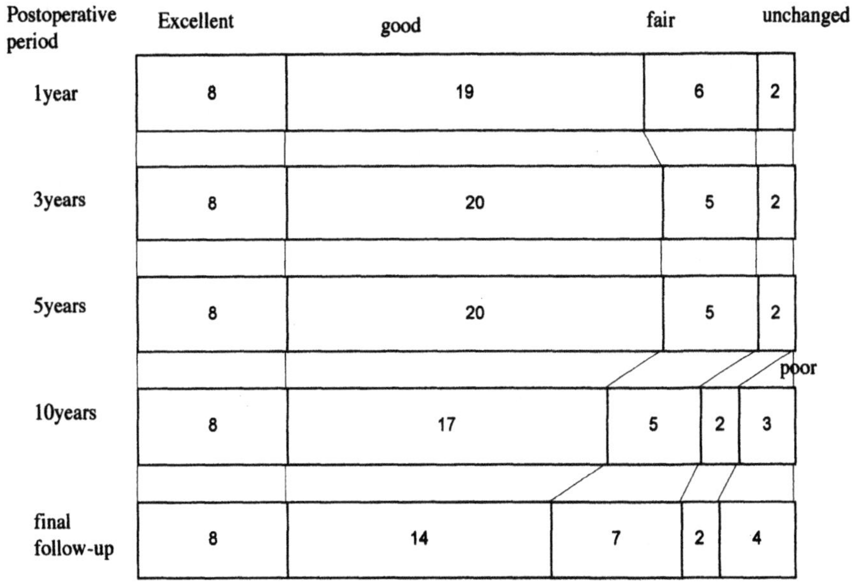

Fig. 13. Changes in the results of surgery, estimated over time by Kurokawa's method, in patients with ossification of the posterior longitudinal ligament who received double-door laminoplasty using autogenous iliac bone grafts

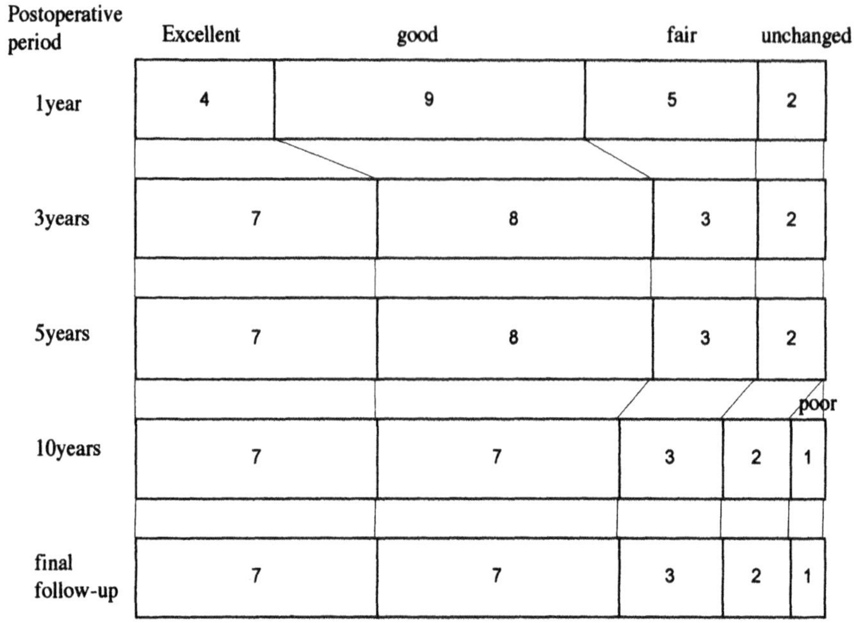

Fig. 14. Changes in the results of surgery, estimated over time by Kurokawa's method, in patients with cervical spondylosis not associated with cerebral palsy who received double-door laminoplasty using autogenous iliac bone grafts

of these 35 patients (72%), the surgical results were maintained until the final follow-up assessment. Ten patients deteriorated neurologically for an average of 8 years (range 5–12 years). Three deteriorated because of thoracic myelopathy from ossification of the yellow ligament of the thoracic spine, which was not directly related to the laminoplasty. Cervical myelopathy became worse in seven patients, and five patients deteriorated after minor trauma (falling down). CT and MRI of these five patients showed residual cord compression by OPLL.

In 18 of the 20 patients with cervical spondylotic myelopathy not associated with cerebral palsy (90%), the surgical results were fair or better 1 year after surgery (Fig. 14). In 19 of the 20 (95%), the short-term results were maintained until the final follow-up assessment. Of the 5 patients with cerebral palsy, 4 had a "good" outcome and one had a "fair" outcome at the 5-year follow-up. However, in 3 of these, cervical myelopathy worsened between 8 and 13 years after surgery. These 5 patients had received double-door laminoplasty combined with posterior multilevel fusion using the long iliac bone. Loss of motion in the midcervical spine because of posterior multilevel fusion was a causative factor of instability of the upper cervical spine, which caused a late deterioration of myelopathy.

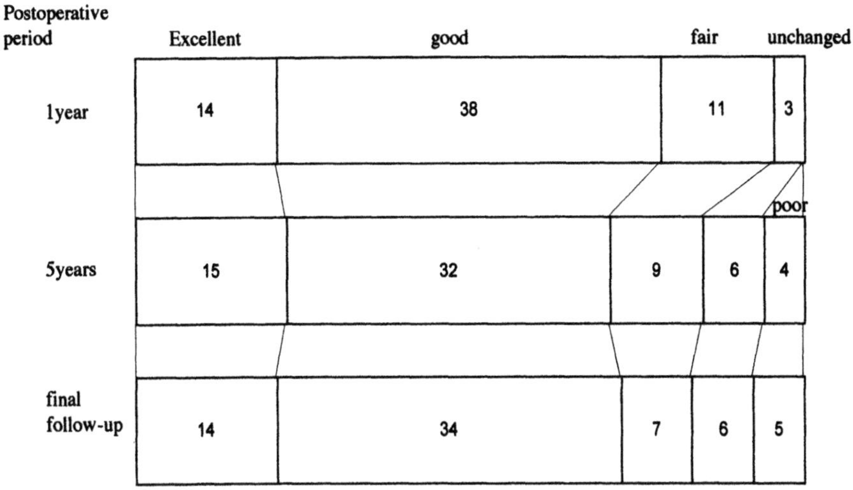

Fig. 15. Changes in the results of surgery, estimated over time by Kurokawa's method, in patients who received double-door laminoplasty using hydroxyapatite spacers

Long-Term Results (Over 5 Years) of Double-Door Laminoplasty Using Hydroxyapatite Spacers

One hundred and four patients with cervical stenotic myelopathy underwent double-door laminoplasty using hydroxyapatite spacers between 1989 and 1995. Patients with cerebral palsy were excluded from this series. The results of surgery were estimated by Kurokawa's method within 1 year after surgery, and 93 patients (89%) were fair or better. Sixty-six patients were followed for 5 years after surgery: 54 men and 12 women, with an average age at surgery of 60 years (range 23–78 years). The average follow-up period was 72 months (range 60–127 months). Of these 66, 36 patients had cervical myelopathy caused by OPLL in the cervical spine, and 30 had cervical spondylotic myelopathy. In 61 of the 66 patients (92%), the short-term results were maintained until the final follow-up assessment (Fig. 15). No recurrence of cervical myelopathy due to failure of the hydroxyapatite spacers occurred. The surgical effects of double-door laminoplasty using hydroxyapatite spacers were considered to be equivalent to those of double-door laminoplasty using autogenous iliac bone grafts.

Surgical Results of Double-Door Laminoplasty in Elderly Patients

The cases of 14 patients (age at surgery ≧75 years) with cervical spondylotic myelopathy, who underwent double-door laminoplasty using hydroxyapatite spacers between 1987 and 1997, were reviewed. There were 11 men and 3 women, and their average age at surgery was 78 years (range 75–85 years); the average follow-up period was 27 months (range 3–96 months). Their surgical results were compared with the results from 17 younger patients, under 50 years of age at surgery, with cervical spondylotic myelopathy who underwent laminoplasty during the same period. These 17 patients included 15 men and 2 women, their average age at surgery was 43 years (range 26–50 years), and the average follow-up period was 62 months (range 12–108 months). In the older group, one patient had an "excellent" outcome, 8 had a "good" outcome, 3 had a "fair" outcome, and 2 had a "no change" outcome. In the younger group, 2 patients had an "excellent" outcome and 15 had a "good" outcome. In 8 patients in the older group (57%) and 14 in the younger group (82%), the postoperative motor score of the upper extremities rose to more than 3. In one patient in the older group (7%) and 11 in the younger group (64%), the postoperative motor score of the lower extremities rose to more than 3. These results show that laminoplasty is effective for elderly people, but the postoperative motor function of their lower extremities is inferior to that of younger people. One causative factor is the severity of preoperative motor dysfunction of the lower extremities in the elderly patients.

Alignment and Range of Motion of the Cervical Spine after Double-Door Laminoplasty

Lateral radiographs of the cervical spine in maximal active flexion, in the neutral position, and in maximal active extension were taken before surgery and at the final follow-up. The curvature of the cervical spine was determined by measuring the angle formed by two lines extending from the posterior borders of the second and seventh cervical bodies in the neutral position (C2/7 angle) [9]. The range of motion (ROM) of the cervical spine was evaluated by the summation of the C2/7 angles in flexion and in extension.

Among 55 patients who received double-door laminoplasty with an autogenous iliac bone graft (not including patients with cerebral palsy) and were followed for 10 years after surgery, the C2/7 angle in the neutral position was smaller after surgery, having decreased from a preoperative average of 27° (from −1° to 47°) to an average of 14°(from −6° to 34°). These results show a postoperative reduction of lordosis of the cervical spine. In three patients, mild kyphosis with a negative C2/7 angle (less than 0°) occurred postoperatively, and their postoperative C2/7 angles were −2°, −3°, and −6°. However, their neurological results estimated by Kurokawa's method were "good". There was one patient with preoperative kyphosis with a C2/7 angle of less than 0° (−1°) and his neurological result was also "good." Among 66 patients who received double-door laminoplasty using hydroxyapatite spacers and who were followed for 5 years after surgery, the C2/7 angle in the neutral position was smaller after surgery, having decreased from a preoperative average of 21° (range −3° to 40°) to an average of 14° (range −30° to 40°). These results also show a postoperative reduction of lordosis of the cervical spine. In two patients, a mild kyphosis with negative C2/7 angles (less than 0°) occurred postoperatively, and their postoperative C2/7 angles were −1° and −4°. However, their neurological results estimated by Kurokawa's method were "good." There were four patients with preoperative kyphosis with C2/7 angles of less than 0° (range −1° to -3°). Their kyphosis progressed after surgery with C2/7 angles between −2° and −10°, but their neurological results were all "good." We conclude that double-door laminoplasty is effective not only in cases with lordosis of the cervical spine, but also in cases with mild kyphosis, and that the aim of double-door laminoplasty, which is to prevent the progression of malalignment, has generally been achieved.

In the 55 patients who received double-door laminoplasty using autogenous iliac bone grafts, the postoperative period of neck immobilization by neck orthosis was more than 8 weeks. The ROM between C2 and C7 decreased from a preoperative average of 41° to 10° at the final follow-up assessment. In the 66 patients who received double-door laminoplasty using hydroxyapatite spacers, the postoperative period of neck immobilization by neck orthosis was only 3–4 weeks, and the ROM between C2 and C7 decreased from a preoperative average of 33° to 16° at the final follow-up assessment. Since 1989, in order to gain a good neurological result without severe loss of cervical spine range of motion, we have shortened the postoperative period of neck immobilization, we have used hydroxyapatite spacers instead of autogenous iliac bone grafts, and we have stopped performing posterior fusion except for patients with severe slippage of the cervical spine. This second phase of double-door laminoplasty has improved the resulting ROM between C2 and C7, although some decrease still occurs.

Conclusion

It has been shown that the positive surgical effects of double-door laminoplasty for cervical myelopathy caused by OPLL and cervical spondylosis have been maintained. Neurological deterioration due to the progression of malalignments such as kyphosis and listhesis occur very rarely. Thus, double-door laminoplasty is a reliable procedure. The surgical effects on severely kyphotic cervical spines are still inconclusive.

References

1. Yonenobu K, Okada K, Fuji T, et al. (1986) Causes of neurological deterioration following surgical treatment of cervical myelopathy. Spine 11:818–823
2. Mikawa Y, Shikata J, Yamamuro T, et al. (1987) Spinal deformity and instability after multilevel cervical laminectomy. Spine 12:6–11
3. Miyazaki K, Kirita Y (1986) Extensive simultaneous multisegmental laminectomy for myelopathy due to the ossification of the posterior longitudinal ligament in the cervical spine. Spine 11:531–542
4. Morimoto T, Okuno S, Nakase H, et al. (1999) Cervical myelopathy due to dynamic compression by the laminectomy membrane: dynamic MR imaging study. J Spinal Dis 12:172–173
5. Kawai S, Sunago K, Doi M, et al. (1988) Cervical laminoplasty (Hattori's method): procedure and follow-up results. Spine 13:1245–1250
6. Hirabayashi K, Miyakawa J, Satomi K, et al. (1982) Operative results and postoperative progression of ossification among patients with ossification of cervical posterior longitudinal ligaments. Spine 6:354–364
7. Hirabayashi K, Watanabe K, Wakano K, et al. (1983) Expansive open-door laminoplasty for cervical spinal stenotic myelopathy. Spine 8:693–699
8. Kurokawa T, Tsuyama N, Tanaka H, et al. (1982) Enlargement of the spinal canal by the sagittal splitting of the spinous processes (in Japanese). Bessatsu Seikeigeka 2:234–240
9. Seichi A, Takeshita K, Nakamura K, et al. (2001) Long-term results of double-door laminoplasty for cervical stenotic myelopathy. Spine 26:1330–1336
10. Hirabayashi S, Kumano K (1999) Contact of hydroxy spacers with split spinous processes in double-door laminoplasty for cervical myelopathy. J Orthop Sci 4:264–268
11. Kurokawa T, Nakamura K, Hoshino Y (1995) On double-door laminoplasty splitting spinous processes for stenosis of the cervical spine (in Japanese). Rinsho Seikeigeka 30:566–571

Part 4
Modified Procedures

Expansive Laminoplasty

SUMIO GOTO[1], MASASHI YAMAZAKI[2], and HIDESHIGE MORIYA[2]

Introduction

Laminoplasty has been performed throughout Japan since the early 1980s as a posterior approach for the treatment of cervical spondylotic myelopathy and ossification of the posterior longitudinal ligament (OPLL), and it has generally been considered to provide a good postoperative outcome. However, a thorough evaluation of the long-term follow-up data over more than 10 years has revealed a considerable number of cases in which the patient has deteriorated, indicating the limitations of surgical improvement even with laminoplasty [1]. To achieve longer-term stability of the spine, we first need to understand fully the mechanism of decompression associated with posterior approaches and associated problems [2], and second we must determine precisely which cases are suitable for posterior or anterior approaches based on the condition of the lesions. In addition, when posterior approaches are selected, we should further select either standard laminoplasty involving the range from the C3 to C7 laminae, or expansive laminoplasty involving the extended range from the C2 to T1 laminae. We should also note that approaches to surgical treatment differ between cervical spondylotic myelopathy and OPLL. In this chapter, we outline (i) the types of laminoplasty that we currently adopt, especially the surgical technique of expansive laminoplasty, (ii) the decompression mechanism of laminoplasty, and (iii) the selection criteria for anterior and posterior approaches.

[1] Department of Orthopaedic Surgery, National Center of Neurology and Psychiatry, Kohnodai Hospital, 1-7-1 Kohnodai, Ichikawa, Chiba 272-8516, Japan
[2] Department of Orthopaedic Surgery, Chiba University School of Medicine, Chiba 260–8670, Japan

Surgical Techniques

Three Types of Laminoplasty—Our Current Choice

As shown in Figs. 1 and 2, we currently use three types of laminoplasty: (i) the Chiba University original type (Fig. 1a, Miyasaka 1978, a very easy technique); (ii) the Toyama University type (Fig. 1b, Itoh, best for stabilizing the laminae); and (iii) the Chiba expansive type (Fig. 2, Goto 1988, preserves the continuity of the expanded lamina and the yellow ligament complex, C2–T1 laminoplasty).

Expansive Laminoplasty

The general procedure for expansive laminoplasty is described below.

Positioning the Patient and Incising the Operative Field

Surgery is performed under general anesthesia. During tracheal intubation, it is important not to extend the cervical spine excessively. The patient is then placed in the prone position, and the head is fixed on the operating table with a three-pin head halter. To remove wrinkles from the skin in the

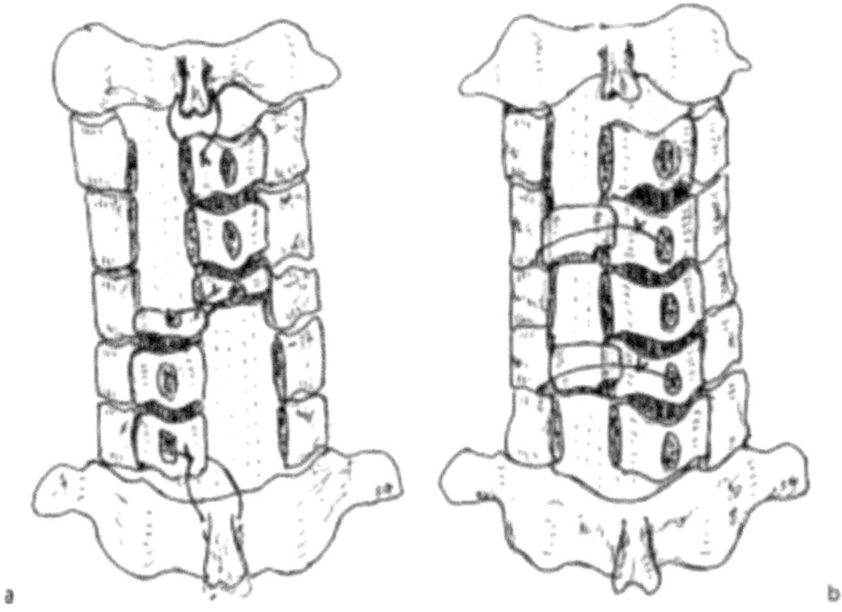

Fig. 1. Laminoplasty. **a** The Chiba University original type. **b** The Toyama University type

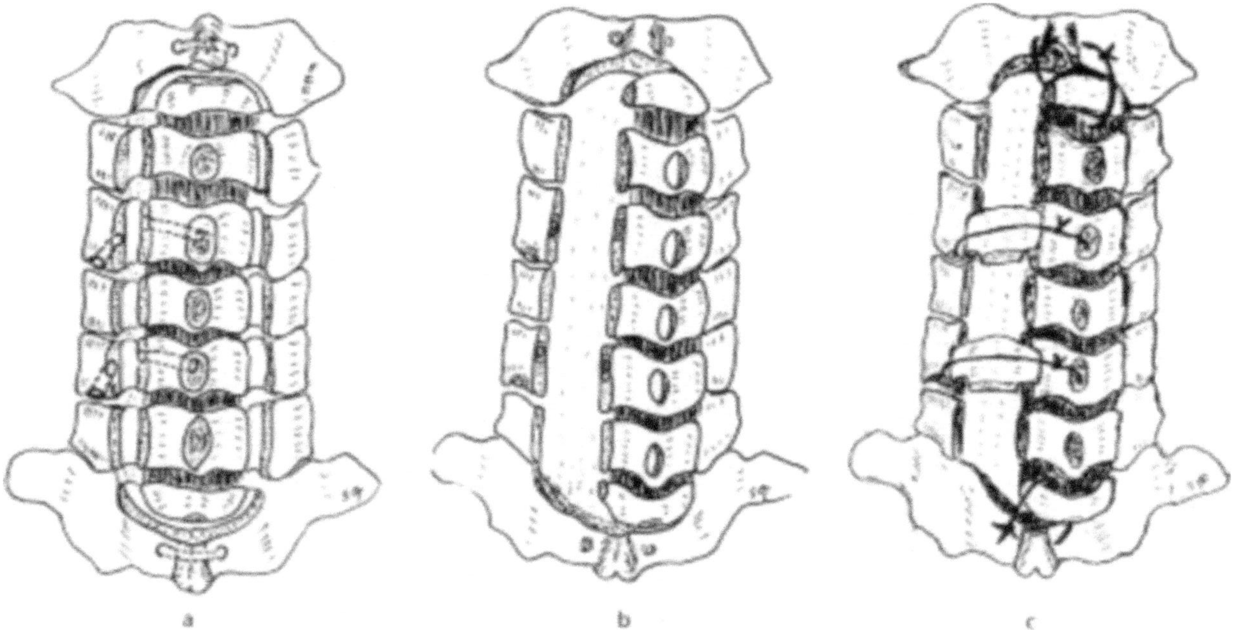

Fig. 2. Laminoplasty: the Chiba expansive type. **a** The transverse troughs (*hatched area*) and tunnels in the C2 and T1 spinous processes (*dotted area*). **b** The elevated lamina flap. **c** The stabilized laminae

incision area, both shoulders are lightly stretched downwards with adhesive bandages, and both arms are placed in the attention position. Following the injection of 1:500 000 diluted epinephrine along the vertical incision line (the midline of the neck), an incision is made through the skin down to the posterior spine from the atlas (3 cm proximal to the inion) to the T2 spinous process. Almost no bleeding occurs when the fascia is incised on the midline. The muscles attached to the laminae, the semispinalis cervicis muscles, and the multifidus muscles are detached to expose the outer edges of both sides of the articular processes. The interspinal muscles in each vertebral space are removed with vertebral pulp forceps, and then the yellow ligament can be seen. After the retractor for the laminectomy is set, the operative field is sterilized.

Making Tunnels in the Laminae

The spinous processes from the C3 to the C7 levels are osteotomized with Liston's knives. A vertical trough is made on each side of the laminae from the lower half of the C2 level through the upper half of the T1 level with an air drill with a 5-mm round steel bur. Transverse troughs are then made in the middle of the C2 and T1 laminae with an air drill with a 4-mm round steel bur, with the ventral cortex preserved (Fig. 2a, hatched area). Tunnels for the passage of threads to tie the bone grafts are then made in the medullary space between the dorsal and ventral cortices of the laminae and in the inferior articular process at the C4 and C6 levels. Tunnels for threads are also made in the C2 and T1 spinous processes (Fig. 2a, dotted area).

Using the diamond air drill with a smaller round bur, the left vertical trough and the two transverse troughs are then drilled until the laminae are cut, and the right vertical trough is thinned until the ventral cortex of each lamina is about half of the original thickness. In this procedure, attention should be paid to bleeding from the epidural venous plexus. The yellow ligament behind the left vertical trough is cut starting from the caudal direction, while the lamina flap is elevated from the open side (the right trough serves as a hinge, Fig. 2b). Two bone blocks made from the resected C5–T1 spinous processes are used as grafts. Each block is placed into the gap between the articular process and the elevated lamina at the C4 and C6 levels, and the laminae are stabilized with the blocks and nylon threads. The elevated part of the C2 and T1 laminae are shifted to the right and sutured to the C2 and T1 spinous processes, respectively (Fig. 2c). In this procedure, if the cervical spine is excessively extended, i.e., the neck is flexed anteriorly, suturing becomes difficult, and therefore the initial position of the patient should be with the neck only slightly flexed posteriorly.

After the operative field has been well cleaned, bone chips are grafted into the right trough (hinged side), and fatty tissue is grafted onto the dura mater

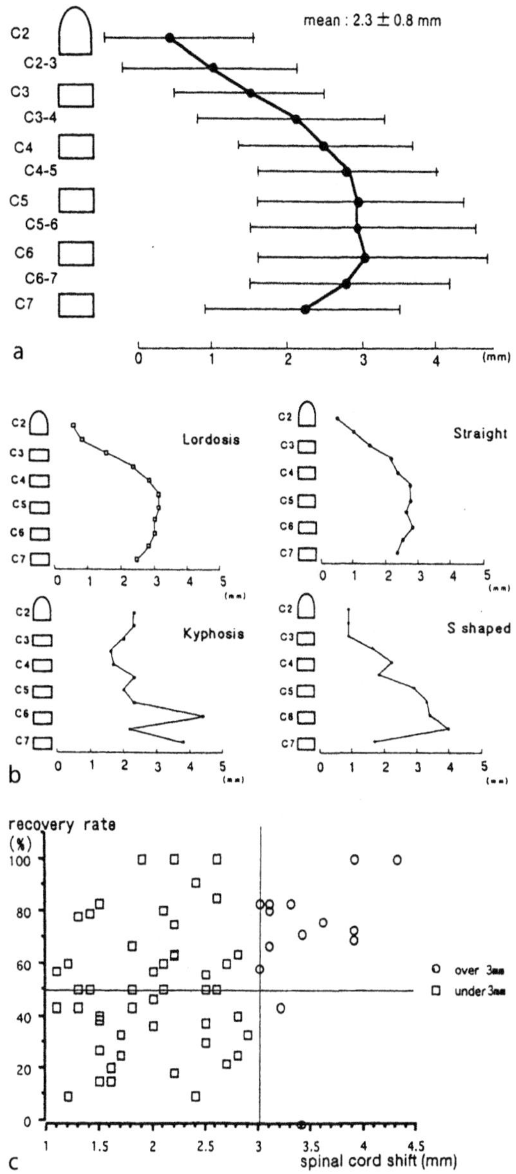

Fig. 3. **a** The spinal cord shift pattern from C2 to C7. The peak shift was 3mm at C6. The spinal cord shift measured 6.6mm at its maximum and 0mm at its minimum, with a mean of 2.3 ± 0.8mm. **b** The mean spinal cord shifts in the different neck alignment groups. In the lordosis group, the peak shift was 3.1mm at C4–C5 and C5. The straight-neck group showed peak shifts of less than 3mm, with a maximum shift of 2.8mm at C6. In the kyphosis and S-shaped groups, the shift was <2mm at C3–C4, C4, and C5; these shifts were less than those in the lordosis and straight-neck groups. **c** Patients with cervical spondylotic myelopathy and ossification of the posterior longitudinal ligament (OPLL) were evaluated to determine their neurological state by examining the recovery rate of their Japanese Orthopaedic Association score. The average recovery rate of patients with a shift of >3mm was 70.4% ± 25.2%, and that of patients with a shift of <3mm was 48.7% ± 23.5%. A significant difference was observed between patients with shift of >3mm and those with a shift of <3mm using the unpaired *t*-test ($P < 0.05$) (From [2])

on the open side to prevent scar formation. A suction drain is set on the laminae, and the field is closed with three-layer sutures.

Mechanism of Decompression in Laminoplasty

Although many different types of laminoplasty have been performed in Japan, all share the common aim of decompression of the spinal cord by posterior shifting of the spinal cord. However, we have found an unexpectedly

Table 1. Selection criteria for surgery for cervical spondylotic myelopathy

- Phase 1 (1960–1968)
  - Smith-Robinson method
- Phase 2 (1968–1980)
  - Single level: Cloward's method
  - Multilevel: subtotal spondylectomy (Inoue's method); removal of the posterior longitudinal ligament
- Phase 3 (1980–1987)
  - Single-level spondylosis or disc herniation: anterior surgery
  - Multilevel spondylosis (within three intervertebral levels)
    - Without a narrow spinal canal[a]: anterior surgery
    - With a narrow spinal canal: posterior surgery (Chiba method)
  - Multilevel spondylosis (over three intervertebral levels): posterior surgery
  - Multilevel disc herniation associated with a narrow spinal canal: combined anterior and posterior surgery
- Phase 4 (1988–present)
  - Single-level spondylosis or disc herniation: anterior surgery
  - Multilevel spondylosis
    - Without a narrow spinal canal: anterior surgery[b]
    - With a narrow spinal canal[c]
      - With marked anterior cord compression: anterior surgery
      - Without marked anterior cord compression: posterior surgery
    - With kyphotic malalignment: anterior surgery
    - With hyperlordotic malalignment: posterior surgery
  - Elderly or poor general condition: posterior surgery

[a] A narrow spinal canal in phase 3 means an anteroposterior (AP) diameter of the bony canal ≤ 11 mm
[b] Anterior surgery in phase 4 means iliac bone grafting within three intervertebral levels. Fibular grafting is used for fusion from C3 to C7
[c] A narrow spinal canal in phase 4 means an AP diameter of the bony canal <13 mm

high percentage of patients with insufficient postoperative neurological recovery. We therefore measured the postoperative cord shift in 65 patients who underwent both pre- and postoperative computed tomography myelography to clarify the optimal decompression area that results in sufficient posterior shift of the cord. In patients who received C3–C7 laminoplasty, the cord shift ranged from a maximum of 6.6 mm to a minimum of 0 mm, with a mean of 2.3 mm (Fig. 3a). The peak shift was 3 mm at C6, and there was no significant difference in shift between the cervical spondylosis and the OPLL groups, but differences were seen based on neck alignment (Fig. 3b). There was a significant difference in the neurological recovery ratio, as evaluated by the Japanese Orthopaedic Association (JOA) scoring system, in patients with a cord shift of over 3 mm compared with those with a shift of less than 3 mm. A mean shift of at least 3 mm was therefore critical for good neurological improvement (Fig. 3c). An upward or downward shift of one level in advanced laminoplasty was related to a significantly larger spinal cord shift in the upper or lower cervical spine, respectively. These results suggest that decompression by laminoplasty was insufficient in patients with massive and adhesive anterior cord compressive factors with kyphotic alignment. Extensive upward and downward decompression by C2–T1 laminoplasty is therefore indicated when the cord compressive factor is on the upper or lower end of the C3 and C7 areas.

Selection Criteria for Posterior and Anterior Approaches

Based on our long-term follow-up studies of patients who received anterior or posterior surgery for the treatment of cervical spondylotic myelopathy [3] and OPLL [4], our current selection criteria for surgery are in phase 4 for both cervical spondylotic myelopathy (Table 1) and OPLL (Table 2 and Fig. 4).

Table 2. Selection criteria and techniques for a surgical approach for OPLL

Phase 1 (1968–1980)	
Anterior surgery:	Single intervertebral disc level: Cloward's method Within three intervertebral disc levels: subtotal with extirpation of OPLL[a]
Posterior surgery:	Multilevel lesion over three intervertebral disc levels: laminectomy
Phase 2 (1980–1986)	
Anterior surgery:	With three intervertebral disc levels: subtotal spondylectomy with extirpation of OPLL[b]
Posterior surgery:	Multilevel lesion over three intervertebral disc levels: laminoplasty (Chiba method)
Phase 3 (1986–1991)	
Anterior surgery:	Cervical distractor and intraoperative ultrasonography introduced
Posterior surgery:	Enlargement laminoplasty (modified Chiba method)[c]
Phase 4 (1991–present)	
Anterior surgery:	Fibular grafting for long fusion introduced[d]
Posterior surgery:	Enlargement laminoplasty (modified Chiba method) for patients with hyperlordotic malalignment, the elderly, or those in poor general condition

OPLL, ossification of the posterior longitudinal ligament

[a] C4 or lower levels

[b] C3 or lower levels

[c] Dome-like enlargement of the C2 lamina and extirpation of the C1 posterior arch if necessary

[d] C2 or lower levels

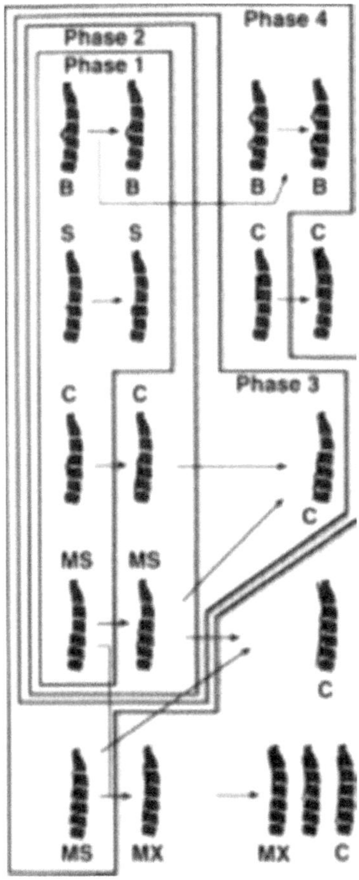

Fig. 4. Classification of the OPLL shape and its natural long-term course. The selection criteria for the anterior approach in technical phases 1–4, based on ossification shapes and distribution types, are shown in numbered boxes. *B*, bridge shape; *S*, single-level segmental shape; *C*, continuous shape; *MS*, multilevel segmental shape; *MX*, mixed shape (combination of bridge or segmental and continuous shapes) (From [4])

Conclusions

We currently use three types of laminoplasty: the Chiba University original type, the Toyama University type, and the Chiba expansive type. The selection criteria for surgical techniques to be used for cervical spondylotic myelopathy and OPLL differ according to the different characteristics of the lesions. Thus, we should bear in mind that the extent of the lesions and the size of the developmental spinal canal are both factors that influence the choice of surgery by either the anterior or the posterior approach, as well as the range of decompression used in each approach.

References

1. Goto S, Mochizuki M, Kita T, et al. (1993) Anterior surgery in four consecutive technical phases for spondylotic myelopathy. Spine 18:1968–1973
2. Sodeyama T, Goto S, Mochizuki M, et al. (1999) Effect of decompression enlargement laminoplasty for posterior shifting of the spinal cord. Spine 24:1527–1531
3. Goto S, Mochizuki M, Watanabe T, et al. (1993) Long-term follow-up study of anterior surgery for cervical spondylotic myelopathy with special reference to the magnetic resonance imaging findings in 52 cases. Clin Orthop 291:142–153
4. Goto S, Kita T (1995) Long-term follow-up evaluation of surgery for ossification of the posterior longitudinal ligament. Spine 20:2247–2256

En Bloc Laminoplasty

Yoshiharu Kato

En bloc laminoplasty, i.e., the insertion of a bone graft between the lamina and the inferior articular process, is widely preferred to laminectomy for the treatment of cervical compression myelopathy. We are now applying a variation for other conditions. This procedure is the true laminoplasty, which was developed from the original en bloc laminoplasty [1] by Itoh and coworkers [2, 3]. It is a type of "open-door laminoplasty" [4, 5], which is generally regarded as a safe and effective procedure.

Advantages of En Bloc Laminoplasty

The advantages of this procedure include (1) reconstruction of the expanded and closed spinal canal with normal tissue to prevent scar tissue (post-laminectomy membrane) invasion, (2) complete bony protection of the spinal cord, (3) it is a safe and simple technique that needs no artificial materials, and (4) easy achievement of the necessary expansion of the spinal canal.

Surgical Techniques

The patient is placed in the prone position with mild neck flexion [3]. Special care is taken to protect the eyes, which must be free from any compression: the Mayfield pin-holder headrest is recommended for this purpose. The neck position is critical because excessive neck flexion may cause massive bleeding from venous congestion while neck extension may cause spinal cord damage. After establishing and securing the proper position, the operating table is tilted up so that the posterior head–neck line is nearly horizontal.

Department of Orthopaedic Surgery, Tokyo Women's Medical University, 8-1 Kawada-cho, Shinjuku-ku, Tokyo 162-8666, Japan

Step 1: Removal of the Spinous Processes

Using a midline incision from C2 to T1, the spinous processes, laminae, and posterior facets are exposed. Each spinous process is cut at the base, as one block, with a Stille's bone-cutting forceps and preserved for bone grafting. Particular care is required in cutting the long C6 and C7 spinous processes to prevent breakage.

Step 2: Making Troughs at the Open Side

An air-drill with a 4-mm oval steel burr is used to create the necessary troughs in the laminae, just at the lateral part of the spinal canal. First, a trough is made at the open side only, to minimize bleeding and to prevent laminar fracture during the subsequent steps. The laminae are usually cut precisely at the medial edge of the inferior articular process. The drill is set perpendicular to the frontal dimension of the spinal canal, and should always be operated from the cranial to the caudal direction (pulling motion) at the maximum speed. It should never be operated in the opposite direction (pushing motion) because of the risk of spinal cord damage if the inner cortex is penetrated. After drilling out the dorsal cortex and cancellous bone, the ivory-colored ventral cortex will be visible. Drilling must be stopped at this depth to preserve the structural strength of the ventral cortex. This is essential for the next step (making the tunnels). Bone wax will stop osseous bleeding from the cut laminar surfaces.

Step 3: Making the Tunnels (Fig. 1a)

The tunnels necessary for passing the nylon threads which tie the grafting bone are made within the lamina and the inferior articular processes, at the open side, from C3 to C7 (or at least C3, C5, and C7). A specially designed awl and pusher (Fig. 2a,b) are used to perforate the lamina. The tunnels are then easily made by manipulating the awl and pusher. After making small holes with the 2-mm round steel burr of the air drill in the inferior articular process, a small bone perforator (Fig. 2c) is used to make the tunnel. The bone perforator must be carefully closed, shaken, and moved from side to side on its axis, but never twisted (so as not to break the inferior articular process).

Step 4: Making Troughs at the Hinged Side

The troughs on the hinged side are made in the same manner, but should be shallower. The thickness of the inner cortex should be carefully maintained to prevent laminar fracture, and to make use of the remaining cortex rebound power.

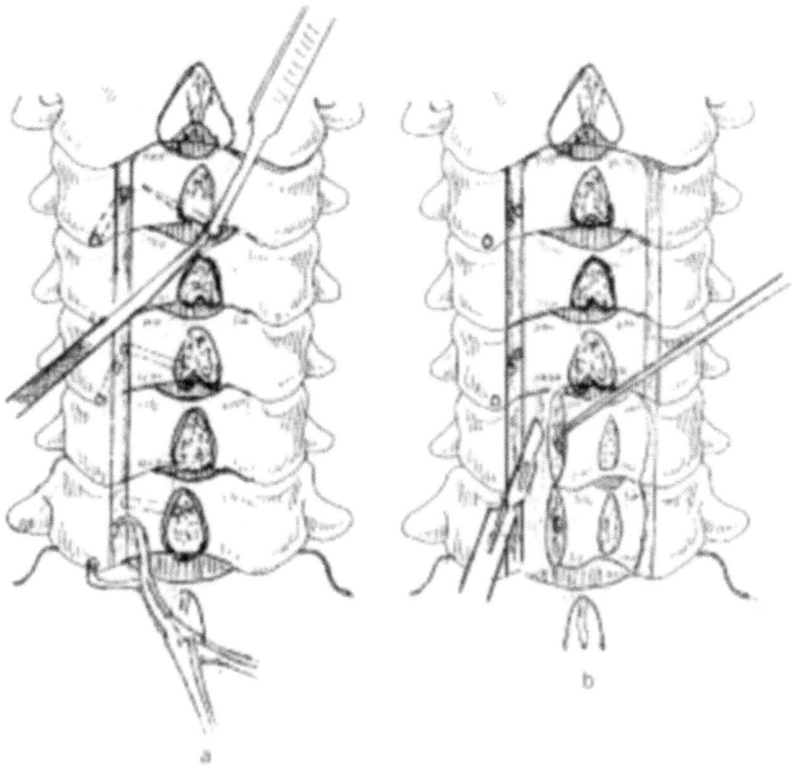

Fig. 1. **a** Making the tunnels. Tunnels to pass the nylon threads through are made within the laminae and the inferior articular processes, at least at C3, C5, and C7, using a specially designed awl, a pusher, and a small bone perforator. **b** Cutting the lamina and the yellow ligament. After cutting the lamina with a diamond bur, the yellow ligament is cut transversely with a scalpel at C7–T1 and C2–3, and longitudinally from C7 to C3

Step 5: Cutting the Lamina and the Yellow Ligament for Decompression on the Open Side (Fig. 1b)

The inner cortex of the lamina on the open side is drilled and thinned with a 3.5-mm oval burr until the underlying yellow ligament is visible. The lamina is then easily cut by gentle, continuous contact with the 2-mm round diamond burr. The maximum thickness of the inner cortex on the hinged side should be maintained to preserve its flexibility and rebound power. The yellow ligament is first cut transversely with a no. 15 small round scalpel at the C7–T1 and C2–3 interlaminar spaces, and longitudinally from C7 to C3, as the laminae are lifted with skin hooks or forceps, allowing the release to be felt by the surgeon as the cut is completed. Occasionally, there may be

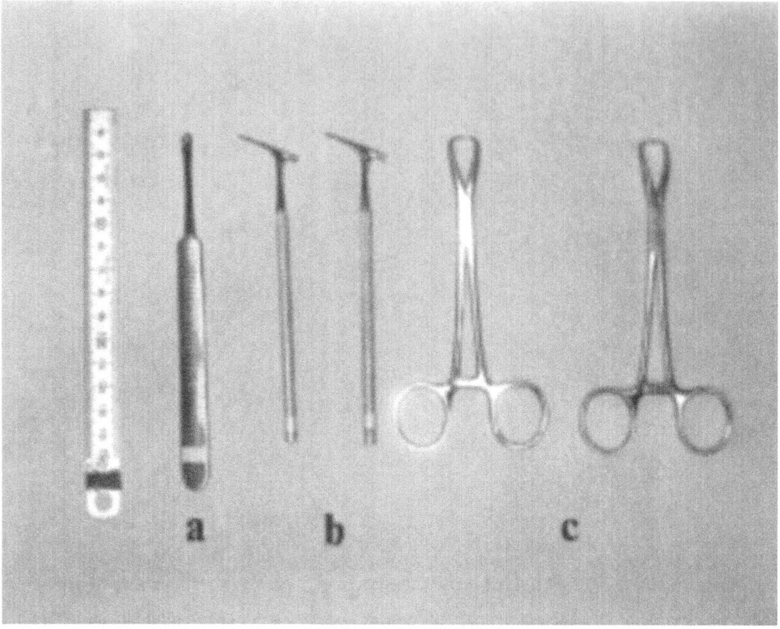

Fig. 2. The specially designed instruments. **a** An awl pusher; **b** a small, sharp awl with a tip angled at 70°; **c** a small bone perforator

significant bleeding from epidural vein, which can be controlled by bipolar coagulation and thrombin-soaked sheets.

Step 6: Stabilization of the Laminae with Bone Blocks and Nylon Threads (Fig. 3)

From the spinous processes removed, three (C3, C5, and C7) to five (C3–7) bone blocks are made, each 8 (C3–4) to 12 (C5–7) mm long, to maintain a 5-mm expansion of the spinal canal. A 2-0 nylon thread is passed through the lamina, the bone block, and the inferior articular process (using a to-and-fro motion with a small needle to pass the thread through the inferior articular process). The bone block is firmly placed into the gap between the elevated lamina and the inferior articular process, and tied with the nylon thread. Finally, pieces of free fat are placed on the dura on the open side, and bone chips are placed in the trough on the hinged side.

Step 7: Closure

Each layer of muscle, ligament (nuchal ligament), and fascia is closed, with particular attention to the secure reattachment of the bilateral rectus major,

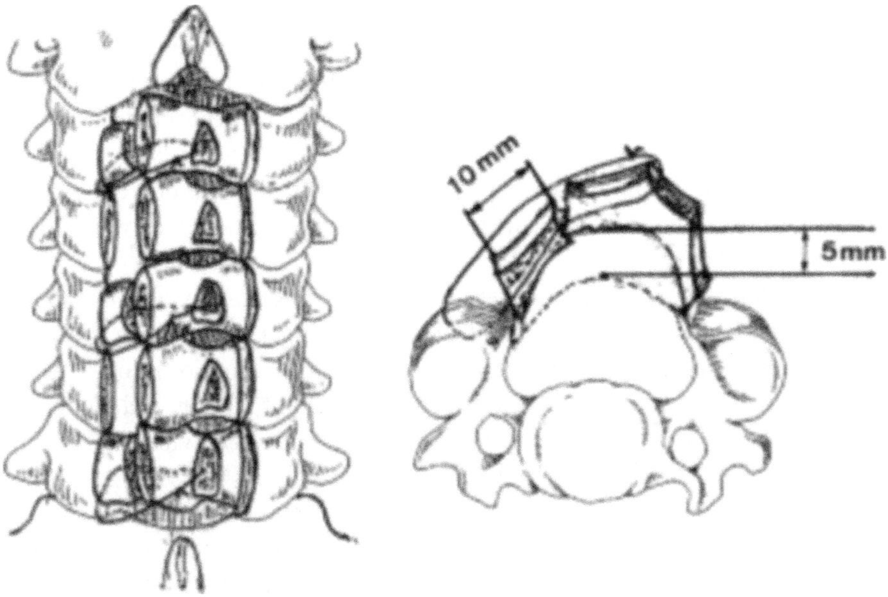

Fig. 3. Stabilization of the lamina. Nylon threads are passed through the holes and tied at C3, C5, and C7 with one bone block in each open gap. Each bone block is 10 mm wide, which results in a 5-mm expansion in the anteroposterior diameter of the canal, and the laminae are stabilized in the expanded position

inferior oblique, and semispinalis cervicis muscles to the tip of the C2 spinous process by suturing.

Step 8: Postoperative Management

A few days after surgery, patients are allowed to sit and walk wearing a Thomas collar. They are advised to wear the collar for 4 weeks after surgery. Isometric neck muscle exercises are begun gradually about 1 month after surgery.

Surgical Results and Outcomes

We assessed 206 en bloc laminoplasty patients who had cervical compression myelopathy. The study patients included 147 men and 59 women, with a mean age of 57.2 years (range 23–83 years) who underwent surgery in our institution from February 1991 to December 1997. They were followed for a minimum of 2 years and an average of 3.3 years (range 2–7.6 years). Their underlying diseases were: cervical spondylotic myelopathy (CSM) only, 141 cases; ossification of the posterior longitudinal ligament (OPLL), 43 cases;

CSM with hemodialysis (HD), 8 cases; cervical spinal canal stenosis (Cx SCS) with disc herniation, 6 cases; cerebral palsy (CP), 4 cases; rheumatoid arthritis (RA), 4 cases. The combination procedures used included: anterior spinal fusion (ASF), 41 cases; partial facetectomy, 15 cases; posterior spinal fusion, 6 cases; an dome laminotomy of C2, 28 cases. The average operating time was 138 min (range 45–225 min), and the average blood loss was 185 cc (range 40–1860 cc).

We rated the pre- and postoperative results using the Japanese Orthopedic Association (JOA) cervical myelopathy scoring system, which includes in the total score upper extremity function (skilled motion), lower extremity function (walking), sensory function, bladder function, and degree of improvement, as well as some X-ray parameters such as cervical alignment, cervical profile angle (Cx angle), and range of motion (Cx ROM) at C2/C7. The mean JOA score for uncomplicated CSM patients increased from 8.9 to 13.3, a 57.6% improvement rate, and for OPLL patients it increased from 9.3 to 14.4, a 63% improvement rate, showing gain in all areas. The improvement in mean JOA scores for patients with SCS and HNP was 64.5%, for those with HD 39.2%, for those with CP 39.2%, and for those with rheumatoid arthritis (RA) 44.8%. All patients improved, but patients with HD, CP, and RA improved the least.

Radiography showed that the average C2/C7 angle had changed from 13.8° to 13.2° in the lateral cervical neutral position. Flexion changed from −10.2° to −3.1°, and extension was reduced from 27.5° to 22.6°. The average reduction in ROM at C2/C7 was 21.4%. Although these results are favorable, patients with HD, CP, and RA had only comparatively fair to poor results.

Complications

Some complications were noted: myelopathy aggravation, 6 cases (acute diffuse spinal cord edema [ADSCE] 4 cases, and epidural hematoma 2 cases); tethered root with monoparesis, 9 cases; wound infection, 2 cases. Two patients who had hemorrhagic disorders developed acute epidural hematoma with quadriparesis; emergency laminectomy resulted in complete recovery. Nine patients had C5,6 tethered root with monoparesis, but recovered within 3 months.

A brief review of ADSCE, which presents as aggravated myelopathy, and its postoperative magnetic resonance imaging (MRI) characteristics is relevant. MRI shows a comparatively wide abnormal change: longitudinally low on T_1-weighted and high on T_2-weighted images (Fig. 4). In this study, serious incomplete paralysis secondary to ADSCE developed in 4 patients (2 men and 2 women) with a mean age of 60.2 years (range 44–80 years). Three of the patients had CSM and one had OPLL, with no underlying dis-

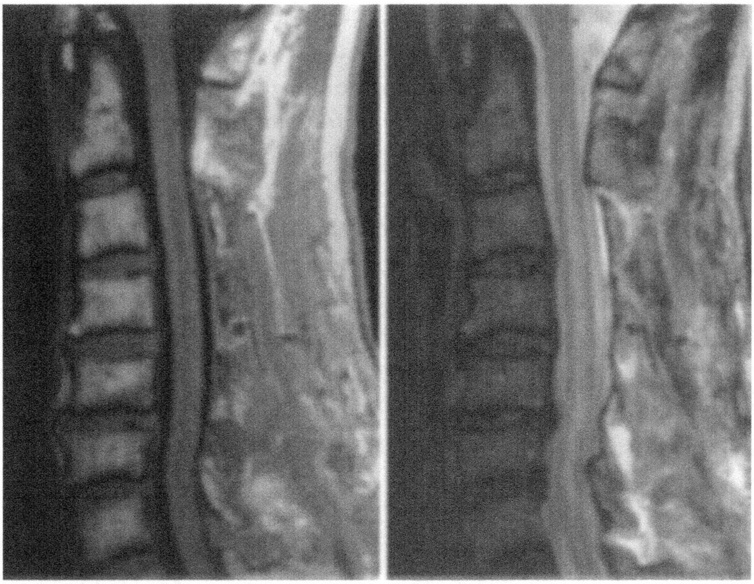

Fig. 4. Acute diffuse spinal cord edema. Postoperative magnetic resonance imaging shows diffuse abnormal high-intensity areas (T_1 low and T_2 high) in the central gray matter on the hinge side

eases. All had C3–7 en bloc laminoplasty alone and the aggravated paralysis appeared immediately after surgery as Brown-Sequard paralysis on the hinge side. However, on the poorer, open side, the symptoms and signs showed improvement. Immediate postoperative MR images all showed diffuse abnormal intensity areas (T_1 low and T_2 high) in the central gray matter on the hinge side, in accordance with the postoperative paralytic site in the spinal cord. Average JOA scores declined from 10.0 to 9.9, with an improvement rate of −1.4%; however, this score had improved to 12.0 (a 29.4% improvement) at follow-up. Three patients involved a kyphotic cervical spine (one patient also had OPLL) and one was lordotic. The MR images of the ADSCE gradually changed to spotty lesions.

Discussion

En bloc laminoplasty is now the optimum treatment for cervical compression myelopathy. Our technique has multiple advantages: reinsertion of the nuchal muscles and ligaments, prevention of kyphosis or listhesis of the cervical spine, shielding of the spinal cord from the pressure of hematoma, and prevention of thick invasive scar tissue subsequent to hematoma [6].

However, there are some risks: the resection of the spinous process and ligaments, which may induce axial pain, and the development of tethered root and ADSCE. The etiology of ADSCE is unknown, but experience shows that the problem occurs on the hinge side of the central gray matter at kyphotic levels. This suggests (1) irregular decompression at the kyphotic level, and (2) reperfusion following the release of chronic compression, i.e., constant chronic compression of the central gray matter followed by rapid decompression, which produces a rapid blood flow change resulting in congestion, infarction, and spinal cord edema with tissue damage in the gray matter.

Increased precision in the use of this procedure is necessary to prevent ADSCE in kyphotic patients. The essential considerations are (1) correct alignment of the instrumentation, (2) the use of combination surgery (ASF, etc.), and (3) insertion of bone blocks of the correct size.

Conclusions

Experience with our series of 206 patients confirms that en bloc laminoplasty is currently the best available treatment for cervical compression myelopathy. We are now working to refine our technique so that we can prevent the major complications of ADSCE.

References

1. Tsuji H (1982) Laminoplasty for patients with compressive myelopathy due to so-called spinal canal stenosis in cervical and thoracic regions. Spine 7:28–34
2. Itoh T, Tsuji H (1985) Technical improvements and results of laminoplasty for compressive myelopathy in the cervical spine. Spine 10:729–736
3. Itoh T, Kato Y (1997) Posterior decompression for cervical ossification of the posterior longitudinal ligament. In: Yonenobu K, Sakou T, Ono K (eds) Ossification of the posterior longitudinal ligament. Springer, Tokyo, pp 143–152
4. Hirabayashi K, Miyagawa J, Satomi K, et al. (1981) Operative results and postoperative progression of ossification among patients with ossification of cervical posterior longitudinal ligament. Spine 6:354–364
5. Hirabayashi K, Watanabe K, Wakano K, et al. (1983) Expansive open-door laminoplasty for cervical spinal stenotic myelopathy. Spine 8:693–699
6. Yonenobu K, Yamamoto T, Ono K (1998) Laminoplasty for myelopathy—indications, results, outcome, and complications. In: Clark CR (ed) The cervical spine, 3rd edn. Lippincott-Raven, Philadelphia, pp 849–864

Bilateral Open-Door Laminoplasty

Hiroaki Iwasaki[1] and Yurito Ueda[2]

Introduction

Cervical laminoplasty has been widely used as an effective surgical treatment for cervical myelopathy caused by cervical spinal stenosis, ossification of the posterior longitudinal ligament (OPLL), and other conditions. Various techniques of cervical laminoplasty are available, and each has its advantages. In 1968, Kirita developed the procedure of extensive simultaneous multisegment laminectomy [1, 2] using a surgical air drill, with the aim of achieving atraumatic decompression of the spinal cord, while Hattori developed Z-shaped laminoplasty [3]in which the lamina was preserved to ensure cervical support and prevent nerve compression by postoperative scarring. Recognizing the varying advantages of these techniques and making good use of their characteristics, we developed bilateral open-door laminoplasty[4–6] as a simpler operative technique in 1977.

Indications

Our technique is indicated for patients with cervical myelopathy due to cervical spinal canal stenosis, cervical spondylosis, or OPLL who require decompression of three or more spinal levels, and for patients with tumors of the cervical spine. In patients with severe radicular syndrome, this technique should be combined with foraminotomy[7].

---

[1] Orthopaedic Surgery, Hattori Memorial Hospital, 4244 Kammaki, Kitakatsuragi, Nara 639-0200, Japan
[2] Department of Orthopaedic Surgery, Nara Medical University, 840 Shijocho, Kashihara, Nara 634-8522, Japan

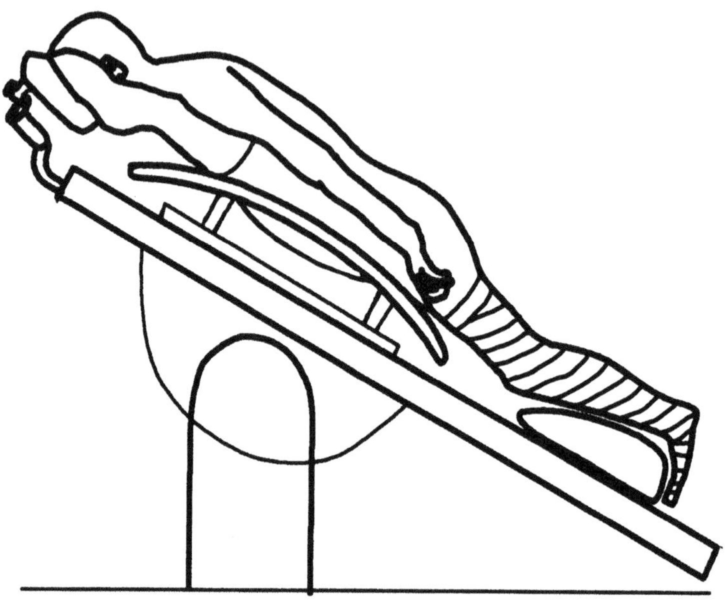

Fig. 1. Patient's position during the operation

Procedure

Position

The patient is placed prone, with the head elevated at an angle of about 30°. Elastic bandages are applied to both lower extremities to prevent hypotension. To prevent the body from sliding down, the knees are extended and the weight is supported using a foot plate. The head is placed on a head holder, and the chest and abdomen are placed on a McKay frame, a Hall frame, or a rolled blanket, so that the intraabdominal pressure is reduced and venous return is not impaired. A plaster of Paris cast is prepared beforehand in order to avoid cervical overextension, which may occur when the patient is placed prone under general anesthesia, and to prevent any abnormal movement of the cervical column during operative manipulation (Fig. 1). This cast extends from the frontal to the precordial region and has a window over the face. It is supported at the metopic and mandibular regions. Pressure on the anterior cervical region may increase bleeding due to congestion, and thus compression should be avoided by placing a spacer such as cast padding on the anterior cervical region during preparation of the cast (Fig. 2).

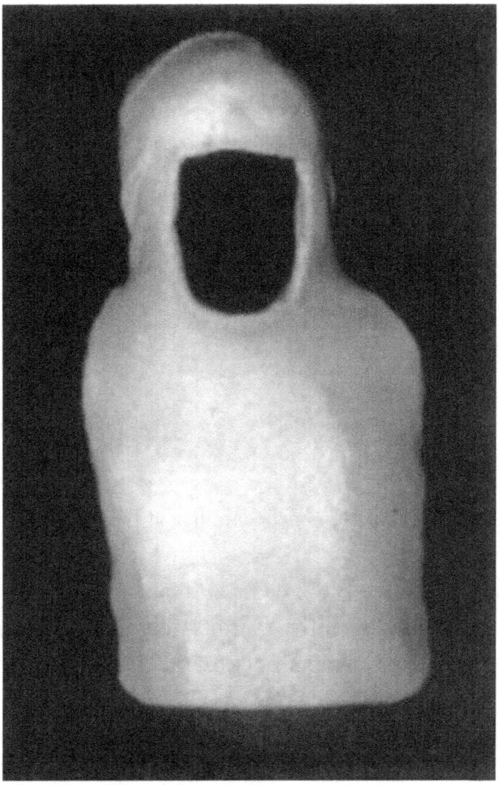

Fig. 2. Example of a cast

Exposure of the Surgical Field

After the spinous processes of C2 and C7 are palpated, an extremely shallow skin incision of the expected length is made as a guide. Then a 200 000-fold dilution of epinephrine is infiltrated subcutaneously and into the muscle layer. An incision is made in the dermis using a scalpel, and is deepened subcutaneously to reach the fascia using a cautery while taking care not to deviate from the center of the nuchal septum. The muscles attaching to the tip of the spinous processes are dissected at the site of contact with the bone. After applying a Gelpi retractor, the paraspinal muscles are dissected subperiosteally from the spinous process and lamina to around the outer margin of the zygapophyseal joint using a Cobb elevator. Dissection of the paraspinal muscles is performed separately for each zygapophyseal joint, and bleeding is controlled each time by compression with gauze while the interlaminar portion of the muscles is left intact. After completion of the dissection, the gauze is removed, and the interlaminar muscle tissue is dissected using Cooper scissors or a cautery. Bleeding during dissection can be

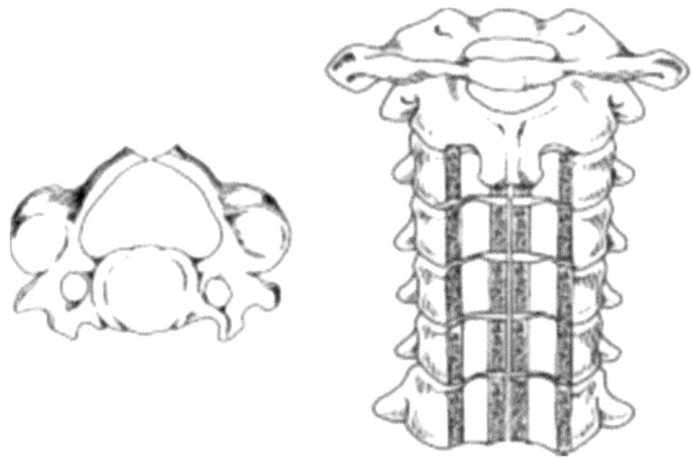

Fig. 3. Dissection of the laminae at the midline

controlled effectively and safely using a bipolar coagulator. The surgical field is exposed using a Beckmann retractor or the like with a blade of the appropriate length.

Resection of the Spinous Processes

After the spinous processes are resected with bone-cutting forceps, the cancellous bone is nipped away using a bone rongeur to expose the ventral cortical bone. At this stage, soft tissues such as the ligamentum flavum are removed sufficiently so that the tip of the air drill is not caught later.

Dissection of the Lamina

After the ventral cortex is cut to a very thin plate of uniform thickness using a spherical diamond bur 4 mm in diameter, the median part of the lamina is dissected from the caudal to the cranial direction with a Davis dissector or a Penfield trepan, or the median part of the arch is directly dissected using a 1.5-mm diamond bur. Direct dissection is done with a small bur, because cutting of the ventral cortex cannot be detected clearly if a large one is used (Fig. 3). Since the lamina of C2 interferes with mobilization of the C3 lamina, dome-shaped dissection of the caudal aspect of the C2 lamina is done beforehand.

Preparation of the Lateral Gutters

The position of the lateral gutters is set so that the inner margin of each gutter corresponds with that of the zygapophyseal joint. Since the cranial and caudal sides of the ventral margin of the lamina are located dorsally and ventrally, respectively, exhibiting a roof-tile-like arrangement, the caudal and cranial sides tend to become too thin and too thick, respectively, if the gutters are of uniform depth. Bearing this in mind, cutting is continued with a 4-mm steel bur until the ventral lamina is exposed, followed by cutting down with a 3-mm diamond bur until mobility of the lamina is obtained. If one is experienced in this procedure, whether mobility has been obtained can be determined from the slight movement of the lamina during lateral gutter preparation. It can be determined easily if the medial margin is pulled up with a Penfield trepan or Davis dissector. To control bleeding during lateral gutter preparation, hemostatic agents such as microfibrillary collagen hydrochloride can be used, or a diamond bur may be employed from the beginning, although the operating time would be slightly increased. If foraminotomy is performed beforehand on all intervertebral foramina, the dorsal position of the vertebral canal can be confirmed, allowing a uniform thickness of ventral cortex to be left, and nerve root decompression can also be performed simultaneously. Foraminotomy can be performed safely if it is started by resecting the boundary between the zygapophyseal joint and the lamina from the dorsal side of the caudal lamina. The foramen is then extended gradually in the craniolateral direction.

Expansion of the Lamina

The most caudal part of the interlaminar ligamentum flavum is cut transversely, and then the laminae are opened to the right and the left bilaterally from the caudal aspect. Since the ligamentum flavum becomes tight in the midline, it is cut using thin scissors. If opening of the lamina is disturbed by a vein, hemostasis is performed using a bipolar coagulator before cutting the vessel. If dome-shaped decompression of C2 has been performed, opening to the right and the left may similarly be accomplished between C2 and C3 (Fig. 4). However, if an inadequate opening is achieved, the ligamentum flavum is also cut transversely between C2 and C3.

When a space forms between the dura mater and the lamina when the lamina is opened widely with forceps, the extent of the opening is judged to be sufficient. However, if the dural sac is opened and no space is seen between the dura mater and the lamina even when the arch is opened widely, the interlaminal ligamentum flavum and the intervertebral articular capsule are sutured with USP 2-0 nylon sutures or similar suture material. Since the problem of loss of expansion usually occurs within 3 months after the operation, it is sufficient for expansion to be maintained during this period and strong support is not considered to be necessary. Next, the paravertebral muscles, nuchal ligament, subcutaneous tissues, and skin

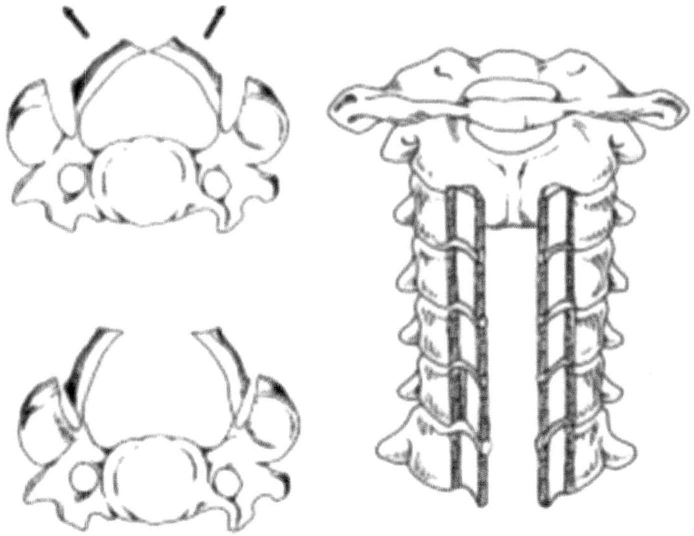

Fig. 4. Expansion of the laminae

are sutured, and finally the wound is closed. Care should be taken during repair of the nuchal ligament so that good alignment is maintained postoperatively.

Postoperative Care

The patient is allowed to sit up after about 1 week of bed rest, and standing and walking are permitted by 1 week after surgery. The patient is instructed to wear a loose polyethylene neck collar as protection. Wearing the collar may be omitted if the patient is extremely obese, since it cannot be expected to be effective under such circumstances.

Results

We performed cervical laminoplasty in 40 patients with cervical spondylotic myelopathy (CMS) between 1977 and 1987. The patients had a mean age of 57.9 years, a mean preoperative value on the Japanese Orthopaedic Association (JOA) scoring system for cervical myelopathy of 9.5, a mean postoperative JOA score of 13.8, and a mean improvement rate of 57.3%. During this period, there were 27 patients with OPLL. They had a mean age of 58 years, a mean preoperative JOA score of 9.0, a mean postoperative JOA score

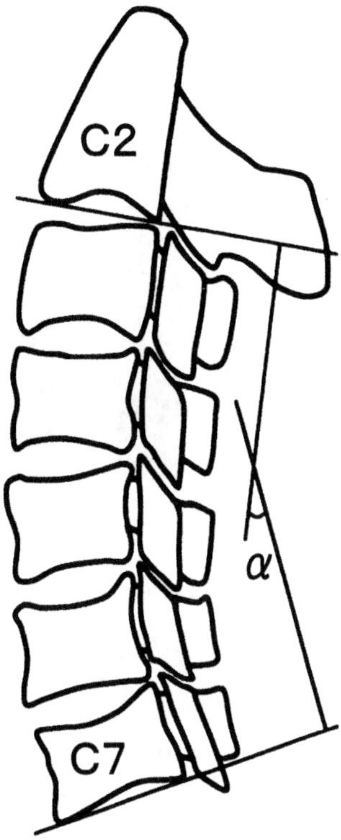

Fig. 5. Measurement of range of motion (ROM)

of 13.9, and a mean improvement rate of 61.3%. For these patients, the operating time ranged from 1h 15min to 4 h 20min (mean 2h 41min), while blood loss was 109 to 1650ml (mean 550m). For 121 patients who were treated between 1987 and 1998, the operating time ranged from 1h 15min to 3h 21min (mean 2h 31min), while blood loss was from 98 to 650ml (mean 304ml). The mean improvement rate in their JOA score was 57.4%. Statistical analysis by the x^2-test did not show any significant difference in operating time or improvement rate between the two groups, but there was a significant difference in blood loss ($P < 0.01$). The reduction of hemorrhage in our recent cases may result from the application of a lower support when creating the plaster bandage that fits the anterior neck.

In patients who were followed up for at least 5 years postoperatively, the range of motion (ROM) of the cervical spine (Fig. 5) decreased to about 76.2% of the preoperative extent at 3 months after surgery, but was 83.8% of the preoperative extent at 1 year postoperatively. Subsequently, it decreased gradually to 75.6% of the preoperative extent at 3 years after surgery, to 74.0% at 5 years, and to about 65.1% from 10 years onwards[8, 9] (Fig. 6).

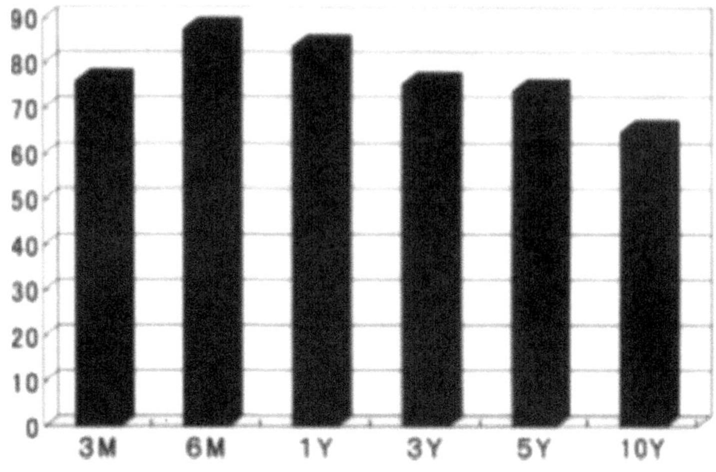

Fig. 6. Postoperative ROM as a percentage of preoperative ROM

Preoperatively, slip of 3.0 mm or more was noted in eight expanded zygapophyseal joints, while it was noted in only two of these joints at the time of final examination and new slip did not develop in any patient. The cervical alignment changed from lordotic to straight or swan-necked in four patients in each case. It did not change to kyphotic in any patient[10, 11].

On lateral X-ray films, the anteroposterior diameter (*a*, Fig. 7) of the lower margin of the vertebral body and the distance (*b*, Fig. 7) from the posterior edge of the vertebral body to the most posterior margin of the expanded lamina were measured immediately after the operation, and again 3 and 6 months and 1 year later, and the *b*/*a* ratios were calculated from these findings. In the CSM group, the *b*/*a* ratio was 0.829, 0.774, and 0.772 immediately after and 3 and 6 months after the operation, respectively. There was a significant difference between immediately after and 3 months after surgery ($P < 0.001$), but there was no such difference between 3 and 6 months after surgery. In the OPLL group, the ratio was 0.913, 0.857, and 0.868, respectively, and showed no significant differences from that in the CSM group. These results indicate that loss of expansion occurred within 3 months of surgery and subsequently showed no further progression in either the CSM or OPLL group. The *b*/*a* ratio at various measurement times was divided by the *b*/*a* ratio immediately after the operation and was then multiplied by 100 to calculate the variation index. This was 92.0 and 94.2 at 3 and 6 months after the operation, respectively, in the CSM group versus 94.1 and 94.2, respectively, in the OPLL group, showing no significant difference between the two groups.

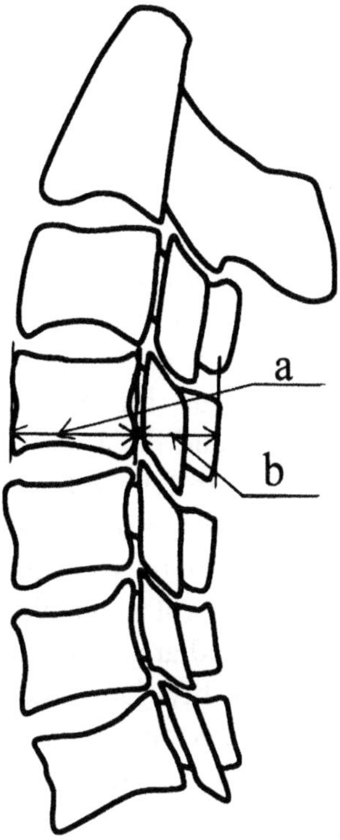

Fig. 7. Measurement of expansion

The clinical results were evaluated using this variation index. In the CMS group, 10 patients had a variation index of less than 88, and 15 patients had an index of 90 or more. Their mean JOA score was 11.0 and 10.1, respectively, before the operation, while it was 14.4 and 13.1, respectively, at 2 months postoperatively, showing no significant difference between the two subgroups. At 2 months after surgery, the mean improvement rate was 57% and 42%, respectively, and was higher in the subgroup with a variation index of less than 88, although the difference was not significant. In the OPLL group, there were 6 patients with an index of less than 88 and 11 patients with an index of 90 or more. Their mean JOA score was 9.7 and 7.9 respectively, before the operation versus 13.8 and 13.2, respectively, at 2 months after surgery, showing no significant difference between the two subgroups. The mean improvement rate was 56.8% and 49.2%, respectively, at 2 months after the operation. In summary, there was little difference in clinical outcome between the CSM and OPLL groups.

Discussion

The beneficial effect of laminectomy for posterior decompression is based on the decompression of nerve tissue by removing compressive factors, including the lamina and the soft tissues such as the ligamentum flavum attached to it. Briefly, this procedure is based on the concept that external compression of the dura mater is caused by the hard tissues alone. It is certain that hard tissues, such as the lamina, zygapophyseal joints, and the pedicles of the arch, are the outermost factors causing compression. If these hard tissues are removed, the paraspinal muscles then compress the nerve tissues and this is exerts extradural pressure. Briefly, laminectomy is performed to release the extradural cavity from hard-tissue compression by the lamina, resulting in the direct transmission of the paraspinal muscle pressure to the dura mater.

In cervical laminoplasty, importance has been attached to maintaining the shape and area of the new lamina, but the compressive force on the space has not been much debated. This indicates that laminoplasty is superior to laminectomy[12] because if a new lamina is formed, compression by the posterior paraspinal muscles will be prevented. Although laminoplasty is reported to have the advantages of less invasiveness and no scar tissue, scarring is observed in the sublaminar space when subsequent operations are performed for tumors etc. However, scar tissue is not observed in the area where the dura mater is in contact with the lamina, and thus optimal expansion may be achieved when the lamina is just in contact with the dura mater.

With our method of cervical laminoplasty, the maintenance of the expansion of the lamina depends on the balance between compression by the paraspinal muscles and the cerebrospinal fluid. Therefore, larger expansion can be gained by making the gutters more lateral (Fig. 8) by the hydraulic effect of the CSF. In, additions loss of expansion tends to occur when kyphotic alignment causes the dural canal to be compressed by contraction of the paraspinal muscles. Since we observed that loss of expansion occurred within 3 months of surgery and did not progress subsequently, the ligamentum flavum and the capsules of the zygapophyseal joints are sutured with 2-0 nylon sutures to maintain expansion for a short period in patients with kyphosis.

The principal cause of loss of expansion is considered to be compression by the paraspinal muscles outside the expanded lamina. It appears that the CSF counteracts such compression and prevents myelopathy. As a result, the influence of loss of expansion was not reflected in the clinical results.

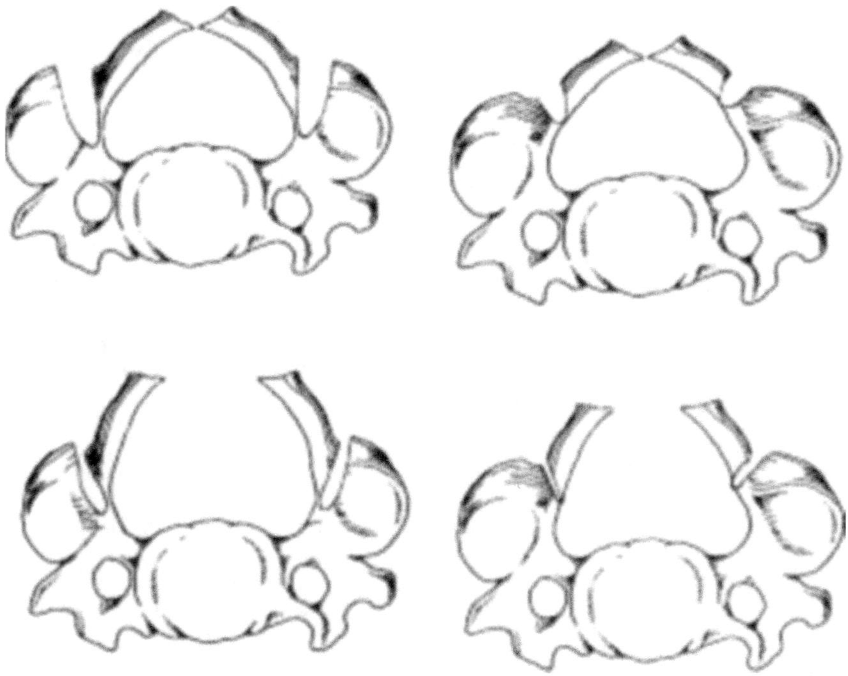

Fig. 8. Changes of expansion depending on the position of the lateral gutters. A larger expansion can be gainred in the lateral portion. *Left*, lateral portion; *right*, medial portion

Coclusions

The following conclusions summarize the results of our investigation.

1. Cervical bilateral open-door laminoplasty has been described, including the indications, procedures, and outcome.
2. Loss of expansion occurred within 3 months of the operation, but did not progress subsequently.
3. The range of cervical mobility decreased gradually to about 50% of the preoperative range over the first 5 years after the operation.
4. This surgical technique is simple and useful.

An example of a case is shown in Fig. 9.

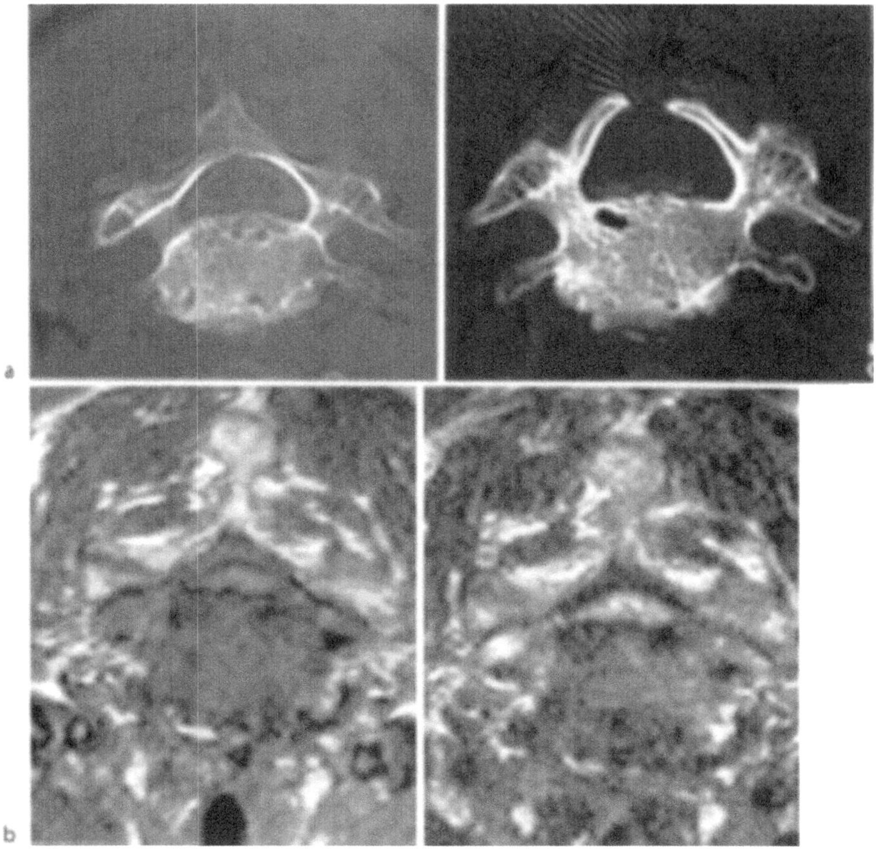

Fig. 9. Example of a case. The patient was a 65-year-old woman. Her Japanese Orthopaedic Association (JOA) score was 9. **a** *Left*, preoperative computed tomography (CT) image; *right*, postoperative image CT image. **b** Preoperative axial magnetic resonance imaging (MRI): *left*, T1W1; *right*, T2W1. **c** Preoperative sagittal MRI: *left*, T1W1; *right*, T2W1. Preoperative MRI showed a marked cord compression at the C3/4 to C6/7 level. The spinal cord was deformed to a triangular shape and had a high intensity area in the T2 weighted MR images at the C5/6 level. The CT myelogram showed a similar cord deformation. **d** Postoperative axial MRI: *left*, T1W1; *right*, T2W1. **e** Postoperative sagittal MRI: *left*, T1W1; *right*, T2W1. Postoperative MRI shows enough decompression of the spinal cord, but also shows that the spinal cord still has a high-intensity area at the C5/6 level in the T2-weighted images. The postoperative JOA score was 13, and the recovery rate was 50%

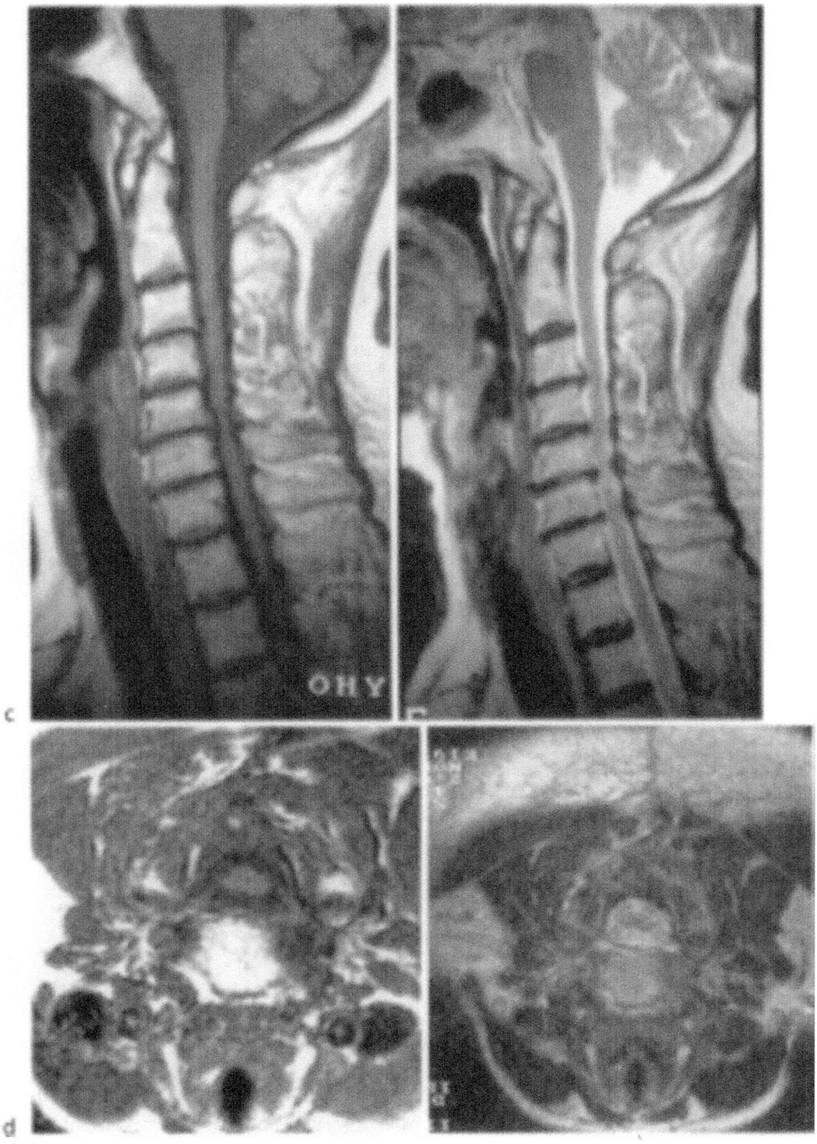

Fig. 9. *Continued*

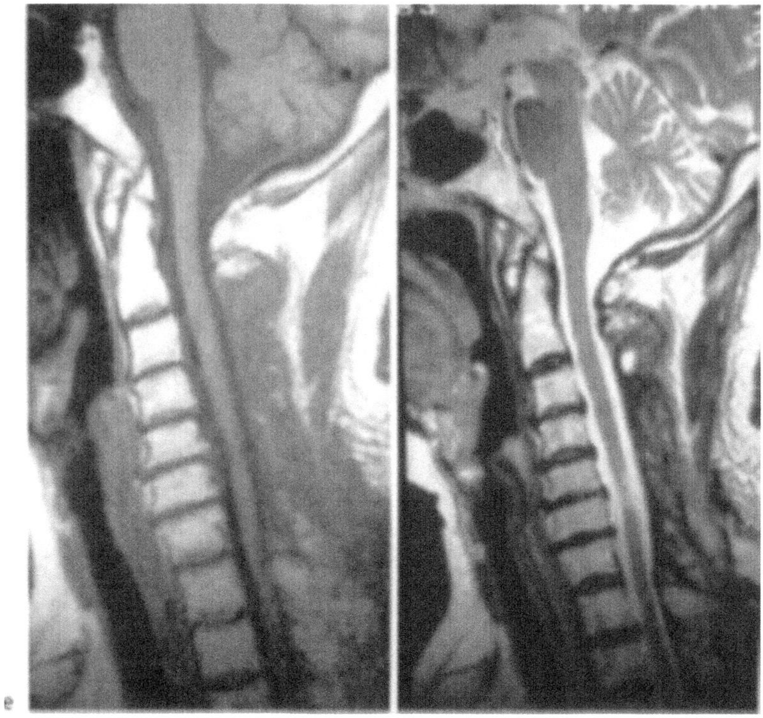

Fig. 9. *Continued*

References

1. Kirita Y (1976) Posterior decompression for cervical myelopathy due to ossified posterior longitudinal ligament (in Japanese). Clin Orthop Surg (Rinsho-seikeigeka) 19:85–93
2. Miyazaki K, Kirita Y (1986) Extensive simultaneous multisegment laminectomy for myelopathy due to the ossification of the posterior longitudinal ligament in the cervical region. Spine 11:531–542
3. Kawai S, Sunago K, Doi K, et al. (1988) Cervical laminoplasty (Hattori's method). Procedure and follow-up results. Spine 13:1245–1250
4. Iwasaki H, Takamiya S, Kambara K, et al. (1980) A trial for cervical laminoplasty (in Japanese). J Jpn Orthop Assoc 54:1238–1239
5. Iwasaki H, Yokota H, Ishii M, et al. (1982) Cervical laminoplasty (in Japanese). Orthop Surg (Bessatu Seikeigeka) 2:228–233
6. Tsuyama N (1984) Ossification of the posterior longitudinal ligament of the spine. Clin Orthop 184:71–84
7. Snow RB, Weiner H (1993) Cervical laminectomy and foraminotomy as surgical treatment of cervical spondylosis: a follow-up study with analysis of failures. J Spinal Disord 6:245–250

8. Baba H, Maezawa Y, Furusawa N, et al. (1995) Flexibility and alignment of the cervical spine after laminoplasty for spondylotic myelopathy. A radiographic study. Int Orthop 19:116–121
9. Okamoto A, Shinomiya K, Furuya K (1995) Reduced neck movement after operations for cervical spondylotic myelopathy. Int Orthop 19:295–297
10. Kimura I, Shingu H, Nasu Y (1995) Long-term follow-up of cervical spondylotic myelopathy treated by canal-expansive laminoplasty. J Bone Joint Surg 77-B:956–961
11. Batzdorf U, Batzdorff A (1988) Analysis of cervical spine curvature in patients with cervical spondylosis. Neurosurgery 22:827–836
12. Tomita K, Nomura S, Umeda S, et al. (1988) Cervical laminoplasty to enlarge the spinal canal in multilevel ossification of the posterior longitudinal ligament with myelopathy. Arch Orthop Trauma Surg 107:148–153

Tension-Band Laminoplasty: A Laminoplasty with Minimal Surgical Intervention to the Spinoligamentous Complex for Better Postoperative Neck Function

NOBUYUKI TSUZUKI, SHIGERU HIRABAYASHI, KUNIO SAIKI, and KYOKO ISHIZUKA

Introduction

The development of surgical techniques for cervical laminoplasty in Japan has shown that the key issue in obtaining better postoperative function of the neck is preserving the integrity of the spinoligamentous (SL) complex in lamina-enlarging procedures [1]. The characteristic structural changes after laminoplasty, namely, loss of lordosis with a mild anterior tilt of the cervical spine accompanied by neck stiffness [2], result from damage to the SL complex. These structural changes produce fatigue in the neck with axial pain, a reduction in the range of motion (ROM) of the neck, and a loss of smoothness in neck movements. All of these dysfunctions cause considerable inconvenience in the activities of daily living [3,4]. The loss of a posterior supporting force by cutting the spinous processes and/or spinous ligaments causes a forward inclination of the neck and the outflow of osteoblastic substances from inside the bone through the exposed bone marrow of the spinous processes and laminae. This might be a major cause of both the stiffness of the healed soft tissue and the posterior segmental fusion between laminae or spinous processes [5]. All these facts indicate that surgical intervention in the SL complex should be minimal for the best possible postoperative neck function. In 1989 [6], we developed a tension-band laminoplasty (TBL) which allowed sufficient spinal cord decompression while maintaining the maximal integrity of the SL complex. In TBL, the tension-band effect of the preserved ligaments allowed early postoperative neck mobilization, facilitated the union of spacers, and prevented postoperative soft tissue contracture. The operative procedures and results are described below.

Department of Orthopaedic Surgery, Saitama Medical Center, Saitama Medical School, 1981 Tsujido, Kamoda, Kawagoe, Saitama 350-8550, Japan

Methods

Principles of Tension-Band Laminoplasty

The lamina is opened in the open-door fashion while preserving the maximal integrity of the SL complex, and a spacer is inserted in the opening. The spacer is held firmly by the tension-band effect of the preserved ligaments together with the elasticity of the lamina. Every neck movement increases the holding force on the spacer by increasing the tension-band effect of the preserved ligaments and facilitates the union of the spacer. Early neck movements prevent contracture of the neck muscles (Fig. 1).

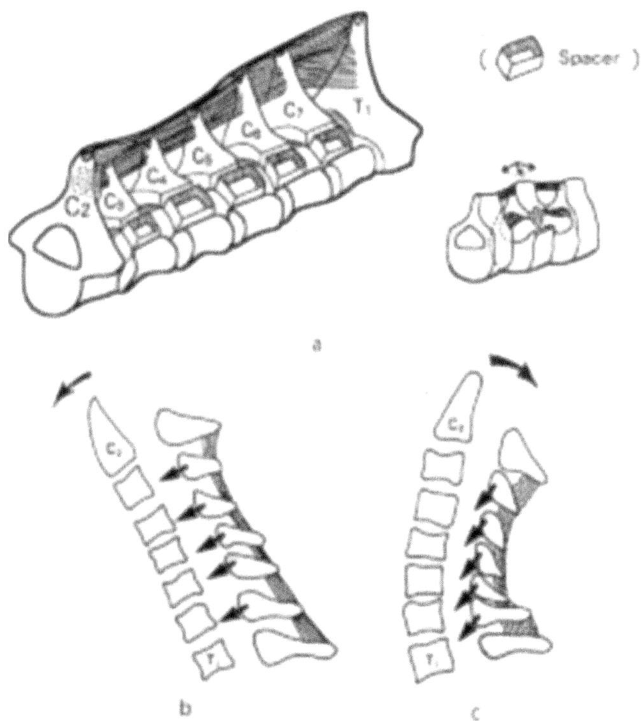

Fig. 1. Principles of tension-band laminoplasty (TBL). **a** General concept. Spacers are inserted into open spaces in the laminae, and then held in place by the compression force generated by the elasticity of the laminae and the tension-band effect of preserved ligaments. **b, c** The tension-band effect of the preserved ligaments increases the spacer–compressive forces in flexion, lateral bending, and rotation of the neck. On extension, the overlapping of the upper lamina on the lower one increases the spacer–compressive forces. Thus, every neck movement stabilizes the spacers further, enabling early neck mobilization even before the union of the spacers

Operative Procedures

Approach

Using a middorsal skin incision, the dorsal aspect of the nuchal ligament and the speculum rhomboideus of the trapezius are exposed. A longitudinal incision is made on each side of the lateral border of the nuchal ligament, just medial to the fascial exits of the cutaneous branches of the dorsal rami of the cervical spinal nerves (Fig. 2a), and deep enough to detach the paravertebral muscles bilaterally from the central structure (Fig. 2b,c). First, the muscles in the superficial layer (the trapezius, the splenius group, the rhomboid, and the serratus posterior superior) are detached from the speculum rhomboideus of the trapezius and the nuchal ligament. Next the middle layer of muscle (the semispinalis capitis) and last the deep layer of muscles (the semispinalis cervicis and the multifidus) are detached from the spinous processes. The interspinous short muscles are left attached. The funicular and lamellar portions of the nuchal ligament are preserved. The supraspinous ligaments below C4 or C5 to T1 are strong and are important for the stability of the cervicothoracic junction and should be preserved. The interspinous ligaments are weak, but the nature of the fibers and their arrangement might be important for smooth movements between spinous processes. Other anatomical structures that should be preserved are the medial branches of the dorsal rami innervating the paravertebral muscles and the facet joints. Detaching the multifidus completely from the facet-joint capsule and too much lateral retraction of the multifidus and the semispinalis cervicis entail the risk of injuring these nerves.

On closure of the wound, it is very important to reattach these muscles tightly in their original places as much as possible. The three layers are reattached in the reverse order of detaching.

Method of Laminar Rotation

Using an air-drill with a steel bur 4 mm in diameter, a shallow longitudinal gutter is made on each side of the lamina–facet junction by whittling off only the outer cortex. On the open side, the gutter is deepened and the bottom of the gutter (i.e., the inner cortex and the lateral portion of the ligamentum flavum) is severed along its length using a diamond bur 4 mm in diameter and a small curette. The spinous processes are then pushed with a finger to rotate the laminae using a lamina spreader as an aid (Fig. 3a). Small trial spacers made of metal are inserted first to hold the laminae open, and then the rest of ligamenta flava on the open side are resected. This resection makes a further opening of the laminae easier. After rotating the lamina to the required extent, trial spacers of the sequired width are inserted into each lamina (Fig. 3b) and fixed with threads.

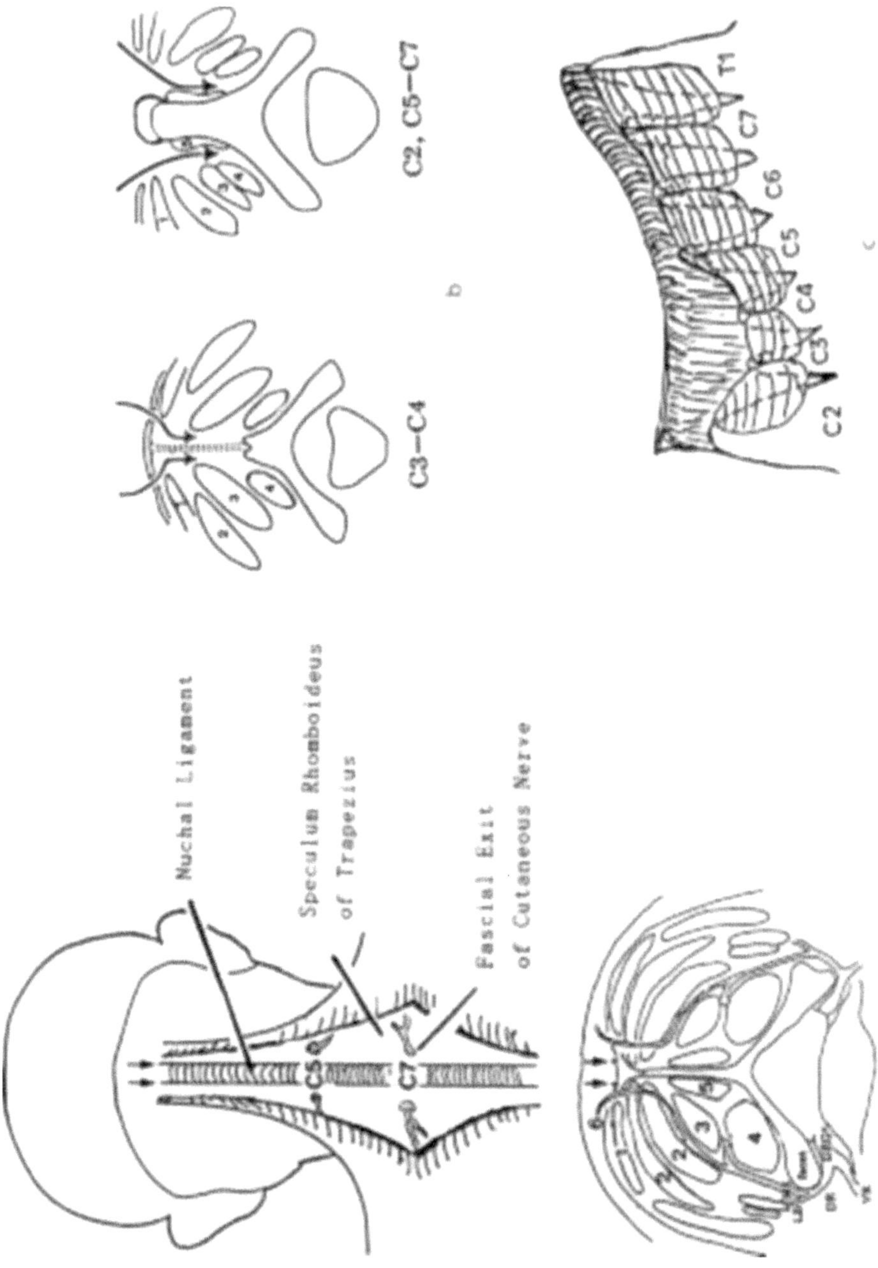
Nuchal Ligament
Speculum Rhomboideus of Trapezius
Fascial Exit of Cutaneous Nerve
C5
C7
a
C3–C4
C2, C5–C7
b
C2
C3
C4
C5
C6
C7
T1
c

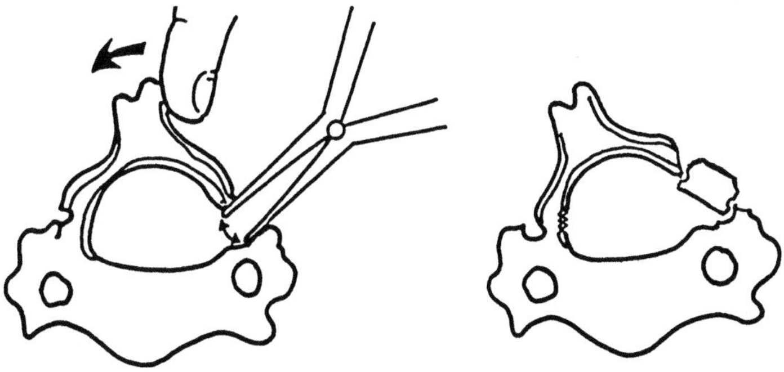

Fig. 3. Rotation of the lamina to enlarge the spinal canal. **a** A bony gutter is made on each side of the lamina-facet junction, without invading the facet joint. Rotation of the lamina is aided using a lamina spreader. **b** A spacer is inserted

Method of Spacer Fixation

A small hole is made on the outer cortex of the laminar and lateral mass edges, and a tunnel is made using the curved tip of a Kirshner wire 1.5 mm diameter (Fig. 4a). A thread is passed through the tunnel and a ceramic spacer of the required width is fixed in place (Fig. 4b). We use Apaceram ceramic spacers (Asahi Optical; bioactive ceramic spacers with a porosity of 40% and widths from 8 to 15 mm are available).

Operative Time and Blood Loss

In cases of C3–C7 enlargement, the operative time is 1 h for exposure of the laminae, 1–2 h for laminar rotation and fixation of the spacers, and 0.5 h for muscle reattachment and wound closure. Blood loss usually ranges from 200 to 500 ml, depending on the degree of venous engorgement in the epidural space.

Complications

Infection occurred in two of 427 cases of TBL performed at the Saitama Medical Center from January 1991 to December 1999. These settled within 6 months with the use of antibiotics and the removal of all ceramic spacers.

Fig. 2. Approach to preserve the spinoligamentous (SL) complex. The nuchal ligament, part of the spectrum rhomboid of the trapezius muscle, is preserved, together with the short interspinous muscles. **a** Lines of incisions (*arrows*) to the lateral borders of the nuchal ligament. Fascial exits of the large cutaneous nerves usually exist between the C5 and C7 spinous process levels. *1*, superficial-layer muscles: trapezius, splenius, rhomboid, serratus. *2*, middle-layer muscle: semispinalis capitis. *3* and *4*, deep-layer muscles: semispinalis cervicis and multifidus. *5*, interspinous muscles. *6*, cutaneous nerve. **b** Muscle detachment at the upper and lower cervical levels. **c** SL complex after completion of the exposure

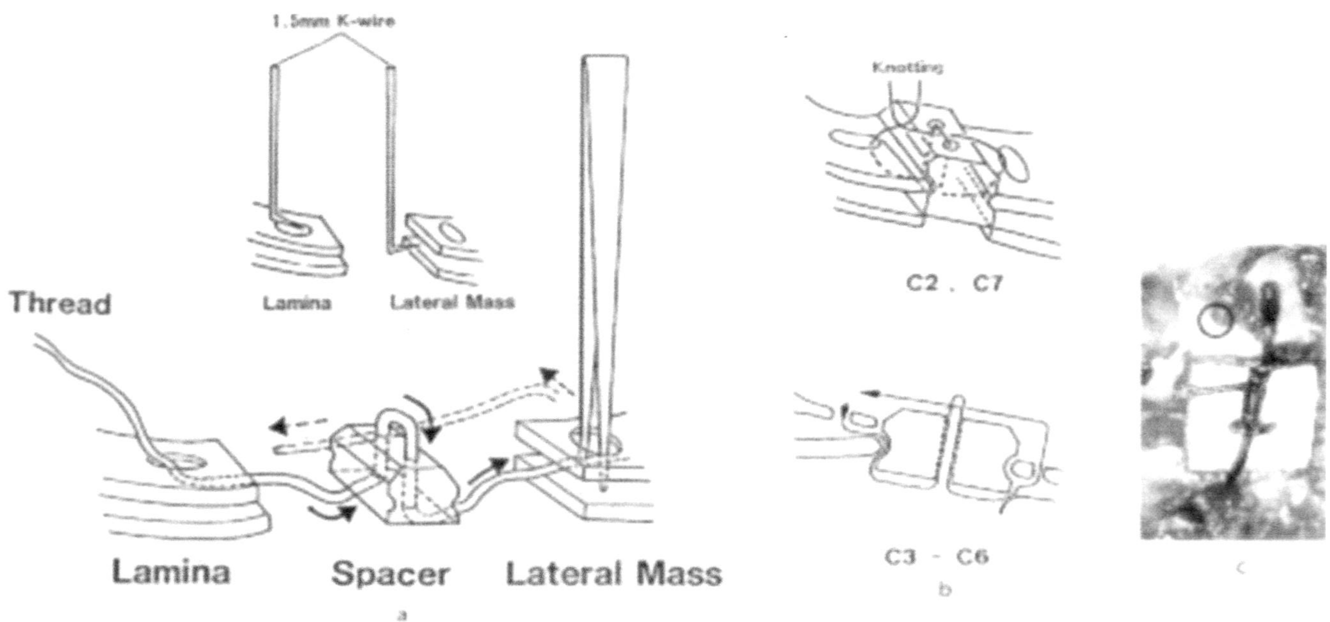

Fig. 4. Method of spacer fixation. **a** A thread, the tip of which is hardened with skin-adhesive material, is passed through the lamina, the spacer, and the lateral mass. In the lamina and lateral mass, a tunnel is made between the outer and inner cortex using the curved tip of a 1.5-mm K-wire. **b** A spacer is fixed with a thread. The medial gutter of the spacer is level with the outer cortex of the lamina in cases with a thick lamina (C2, C7), and with the inner cortex of the lamina in cases with a thin lamina (C3–C6). **c** Operative photograph of the fixation of a spacer to the C6 lamina (*circle*)

Infection usually became evident 2 or 3 weeks after surgery, and removal of the spacers was carried out a further 4 weeks later. By this time, the gutter on the hinge side had become stable enough to maintain the laminar enlargement, so that enlargement of the canal was maintained even after the removal of the spacers. After removal of the spacers, the laminar spaces were filled with new bone spontaneously, which formed new bony neural arches within 1 year. Transient C5 palsies occurred in two cases.

Postoperative Management

On the day following the operation, if their general condition is satisfactory, patients are allowed to sit on the bed wearing a soft neck-collar, and on the second postoperative day they are allowed to walk. Active neck movements in all directions are started 1 week after the operation while taking off the neck-collar during the exercises. The neck-collar is discarded completely 3 months after the operation.

Methods of Neurological Evaluation

The Japanese Orthopaedic Association (JOA) score (Table 1) was used for neurological evaluation.

Results

Two studies have been carried out on the results of TBL for cervical spondylotic myelopathy (CSM) and cervical ossification of the posterior longitudinal ligament (OPLL) myelopathy, the first in 1996 [6] and the second in 2000 [7]. These assessed the degree of neurological improvement, the change in cervical alignment, and the degree of preservation of the ROM of the neck. The results for CSM were as follows: neurological improvements (pre-/postoperative mean JOA scores) were 10.1/14.4 and 10.4/12.9, and mean preservation ratios of ROM were 79% and 60% of preoperative ROM, for the first and second studies, respectively. No postoperative changes in the mean alignment of the cervical spine in the neutral position were found in either study. In some cases, including those with small OPLL, some improvements in ROM were noted postoperatively (Fig. 5). Regarding spacer stability, new bone formation between the lamina and the ceramic spacer was visible to some extent in 64% of patients 4–6 months after the operation. No absorption of the spacers was observed. Dislocation of the spacers occurred in 0.3% of those inserted (2/590) due to loose fixation, but these were left in place because they did not impinge on the spinal cord or the spinal nerves.

A questionnaire study of postoperative axial symptoms was undertaken in 1999 [8] by a rehabilitation team which did not include any orthopedic

Table 1. Japanese Orthopaedic Association (JOA) score for the evaluation of cervical myelopathy

1. Motor function
Upper extremity
Feeding oneself with chopsticks or a spoon
(0) Total disturbance: unable to feed oneself
(1) Severe disturbance: unable to handle chopsticks, but able to handle a spoon
(2) Moderate disturbance in the use of chopsticks
(3) Mild disturbance in the use of chopsticks
(4) Normal
Lower extremity
Gait
(0) Total disturbance: unable to walk
(1) Severe disturbance: needs aid on a flat floor
(2) Moderate disturbance: needs aid on stairs
(3) Mild disturbance: needs no aid on stairs, but unstable
(4) Normal
2. Sensory function
Upper extremity, lower extremity, trunk
(0) Apparent sensory loss or paresthesia
(1) Mild sensory loss or paresthesia
(2) Normal
3. Bladder function
(0) Total disturbance: complete retention or incontinence
(1) Severe disturbance: incomplete retention, incomplete incontinence or straining
(2) Mild disturbance: frequency or hesitation
(3) Normal

physicians who had been involved in the surgery. Sixty-two patients took part (53 men and 9 women), including both CSM and OPLL. In all cases the postoperative period was more than 1 year. Thirty-four patients (55%) felt some restriction of neck ROM and 74% had some axial complaints. Twenty-eight patients (45%) felt no ROM restriction, but 71% had axial complaints of a minor nature. Fourteen patients (23%) had some restriction in the activities of daily life, and 14 patients (23%) had some problems in their work-related activities. The mean JOA score of patients with positive axial complaints was 13.9, and that of patients with negative axial complaints was 15.8. The difference between them was statistically significant ($P = 0.05$).

Discussion

Laminoplasties which destroy the SL complex result in a loss of cervical lordosis, with a tendency for the spine to become straight or to acquire an anterior tilt of 8–10° on average, and with postoperative ROM being restricted to 40%–60% of the patient's original ROM [9]. TBL gave better results, sug-

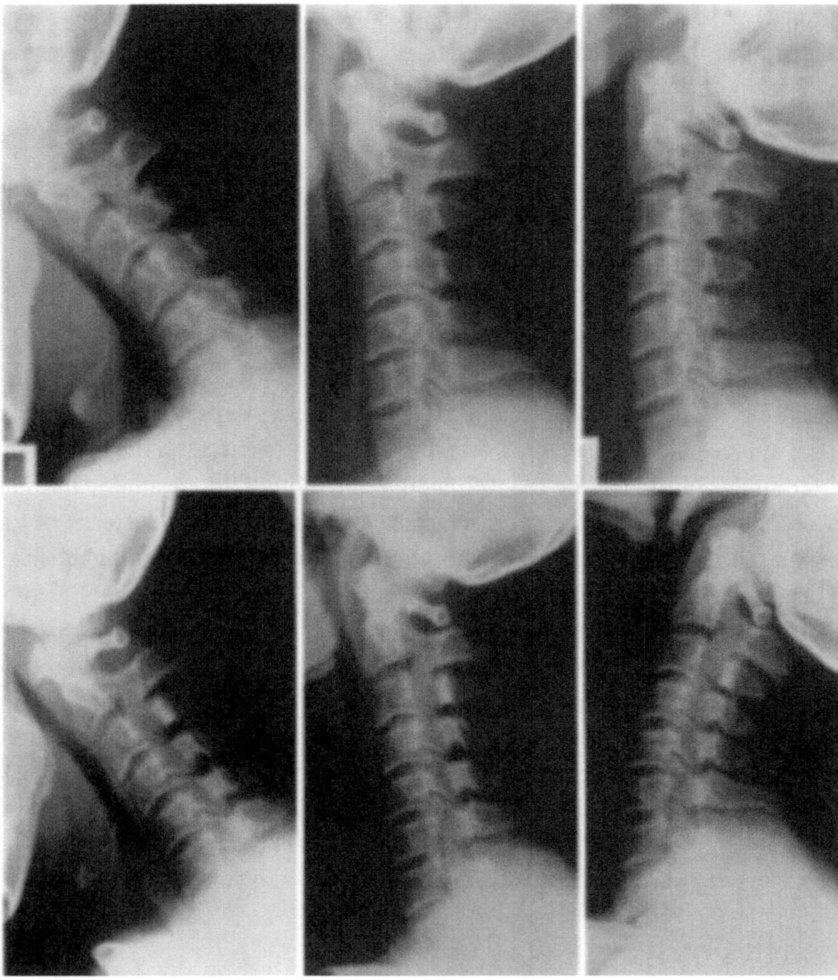

Fig. 5. Radiographs after TBL. Male, 46 years old, with a small segmental ossification of the posterior longitudinal ligament (OPLL) at C5. Result after 4 years. **a** Preoperative and **b** postoperative lateral radiograms. *Left*, flexion; *center*, neutral; *right*, extension. Postoperatively, no axial symptoms were present and the extension of the neck was clearly improved, while the flexion and the neutral alignment of the neck were almost unchanged. Pre-/postoperative Japanese Orthopaedic Association scores were 14/17 (full recovery)

gesting that preservation of the integrity of the SL complex might be important for better postoperative neck function. However, an exact controlled trial has not yet been done, and therefore the full significance of preserving the SL complex awaits further study.

For postoperative axial symptoms such as pain, stiffness, and excessive fatigue of the neck–shoulder complex there is no reliable method of evaluation. The nature of axial symptoms is subjective, and in almost all previous studies the evaluation of the degree of axial symptoms was performed by a team of observers which included the surgeons, and therefore the data lacked reliability. Our questionnaire study was performed by physicians who had not been involved in the surgery, and showed a high percentage of axial complaints even from patients whose necks moved well. An interesting result was that patients with lower recovery scores complained more of postoperative axial symptoms than those with higher recovery scores, even if the operative procedures carried out were identical. This implies that the postoperative axial symptoms have two components, one produced by the surgical intervention and the other by the residual preoperative axial symptoms. This fact should be considered in all future studies of postoperative axial symptoms. Experience shows that severe or moderate axial symptoms after laminoplasty can be relieved by the injection of an anesthetic into the posterior branches of the cervical spinal nerves, and by an increase in the power of the neck-stabilizing muscles and the shoulder-suspending muscles. This indicates that in patients with a postoperative increase in axial complaints, irritation of the posterior branches of the cervical spinal nerves caused by the structural changes made during the operation might be playing a role to a greater or lesser extent. Inevitable slight or mild axial symptoms after cervical laminoplasty are pain or an unpleasant feeling in the neck and shoulder. These symptoms are caused by extensive muscle adhesion to the posterior aspect of the cervical spine due to the extensive stripping of the neck muscles in the posterior approach. Therefore, all patients who undergo laminoplasty have some axial symptoms.

Conclusions

1. TBL, which preserves the SL complex, results in better postoperative neck function than laminoplasties which destroy the SL complex, while neurological improvements are similar.
2. After TBL, almost 70% of patients had postoperative axial complaints, some of which were mild. Postoperative axial symptoms had two components, one from the surgical intervention and the other from the residual effects of their preoperative symptoms. This fact should be considered in analyses of postoperative axial complains.

References

1. Tsuzuki N (2000) Problems related to the posterior decompression of the cervical spinal cord for cervical myelopathy, mainly from the results of cervical laminoplasty. J Jpn Orthop Assoc 74:1–10

2. Ishihara H, Matsui T, Kawaguchi Z, et al. (1998) Kyphotic change of the cervical spine alignment after en bloc laminoplasty. An analysis of the factors involved. Cent Jpn J Orthop Traumatol 41:1075–1076
3. Hosono N, Yonenobu K, Ono K (1996) Neck and shoulder pain after laminectomy. Spine 21:1969–1973
4. Okamoto A, Shinomiya K, Furuya K (1995) Reduced neck movements after operations for cervical spondylotic myelopathy. Int Orthop (SICOT) 19:295–297
5. Takeuchi N, Osawa Y, Itoh H, et al. Long-term results of expansive open-door laminoplasty. A follow-up study over seven years. J Jpn Orthop Assoc 70;3:S604
6. Tsuzuki N, Abe R, Saiki K, et al. (1996) Tension-band laminoplasty. Int Orthop (SICOT) 20:275–284
7. Saiki K, Horie T, Ishizuka K, et al. (2000) Relationship between the postoperative neurological outcome and the postoperative spinal alignment in patients who underwent tension-band laminoplasties for cervical myelopathy. J East Jpn Orthop Traumatol 12:233
8. Takahashi K, Suyama T, Tsuzuki N (1999) Postoperative activities of daily living and cervical symptoms in tension-band cervical laminoplasty. J Jpn Orthop Assoc 73:S727
9. Aida I, Yabuki T, Hayashi K, et al. (1995) Long-term results of cervical laminoplasty using spinous processes as bone blocks. Seikeigeka 46:1161–1166

Midline Spinous Process Splitting Laminoplasty Using Hydroxyapatite Spacers

Kazumasa Ueyama, Seiko Harata, Akihiro Okada, Naoki Echigoya, and Toru Yokoyama

Introduction

Posterior decompression and reconstruction of the cervical spinal canal is a common treatment for cervical myelopathy. Since laminoplasty by midline splitting of the spinous processes was reported by Kurokawa in 1982 [1], we have used this method to treat cervical myelopathy due to spondylotic changes or ossification of the posterior longitudinal ligament (OPLL). Since 1986, we have used hydroxyapatite (HA) interspinous spacers instead of an iliac bone graft to maintain the enlargement of the cervical spinal canal [2]. There have been no problems with dislocation of the HA spacers, and good fusion has been achieved. The use of HA spacers eliminates the problems of buttock pain caused by harvesting autogenous bone from the posterior ilium. It also shortens the operating time, reduces intraoperative blood loss, and improves the range of motion below C2/3. Since 1995, we have also used a wire thread saw (T-saw) instead of an airtome for the splitting process.

Indications and Contraindications

Indications for surgery are multisegmental cervical spondylosis with a narrow canal, OPLL with continuous or mixed-type stenosis, and developmental spinal canal stenosis. Patients with a Japanese Orthopaedic Association (JOA) score below 13/17 are recommended for surgery, but cervical kyphotic deformity, soft-disc hernia, and single- or double-level spondylosis without developmental canal stenosis are contraindications for the posterior approach [3].

Department of Orthopedic Surgery, Hirosaki University, 5 Zaifu-cho, Hirosaki 036-8562, Japan

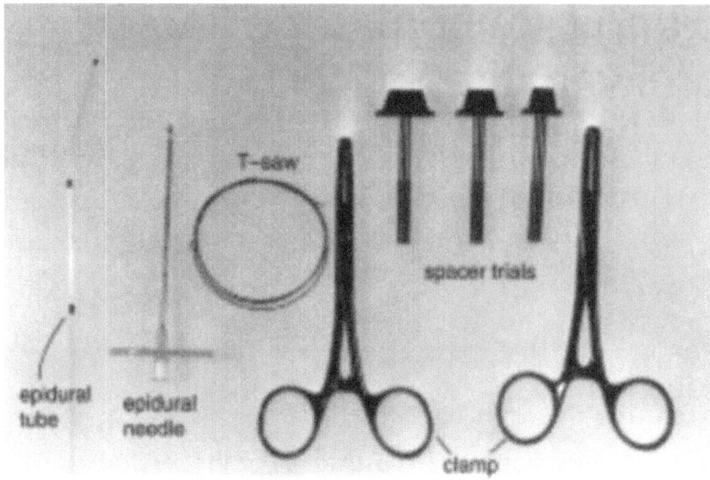

Fig. 1. Operative instruments. *Left* to *right*: epidural tube; epidural needle; T-saw (0.56 mm × 700 mm); T-saw clamp; trial spacers (20 mm, 15 mm, or 12 mm); clamp

Surgical Instruments

A Tuoky epidural needle (16 gauge) (Terumo, Tokyo, Japan) and an epidural tube are necessary for insertion of the T-saw (Koshiaya, Kanazawa, Japan). The diameter of the T-saw should be 0.54 mm. A pair of saw clamps and a device for maintaining cervical lordosis are useful during the splitting of the spinous processes. The porous rate of the HA spacer (Apaceram, Asahi Optical, Tokyo, Japan) is 40%, and there are three widths: 12 mm, 15 mm, and 20 mm. The appropriate size is decided in a spacer trial (Fig. 1).

Surgical Procedure

Preoperative Plan

The extent of laminoplasty is usually from C3 to C7, but in the case of a narrow canal at the C2 level, this level should also be included. If segmental instability is recognized preoperatively, autogenous iliac bone grafting instead a HA spacer is recommended for stabilization.

Positioning

Under general anesthesia, the patient is placed prone on a four-point supporting frame to prevent high abdominal pressure. Mayfield's Tong headholder is a safe and useful device to maintain cervical alignment with a slight extension. If intradural scar formation and adhesion are diagnosed preoperatively in cases which need a second operation, the neutral position is better than the extension position because it will be necessary to use an airtome instead of a T-saw to split the spinous processes. The alignment of the cervical spine should be checked by X-ray before skin incision.

Skin Incision

A midline incision is usually made from the C2 to the Th1 spinous process after injecting the skin with normal saline and 50×10^4 epinephrine. The ligament nuchae is dissected along the midline.

Exposure of the Laminae

The paravertebral muscles are subperiosteally stripped from the spinous processes and the laminae from C2 to Th1 using an electric cauterizing instrument, a Cobb's elevator, and scissors. The semispinal muscles inserted to the C2 lamina are tagged bilaterally with black silk. The edge of each spinous process is cut, and the long spinous processes of C6 and C7 are cut without fracturing the lamina. The interlaminal soft tissues from C2/3 to C7/Th1 are removed with a rongeur, and the yellow ligament is exposed at each level.

Midline Splitting of the Spinous Process

The epidural space of C2/3 is exposed by removing the yellow ligament with an air drill or Kerrison rongeur. A cervical intervertebral spreader is useful for exposing the epidural space of C7/Th1. After spreading the C7/Th1 interlaminal space, the midline slit of the yellow ligament can be found. This is easily removed from the slit with a 3-0 curette to prepare for the entry of the T-saw. The length of the epidural guide tube should be the distance from C7/Th1 to C2/3. The guide tube for the T-saw is introduced through a 16-gauge epidural needle at C7/Th1, and is advanced through spinal canal until it exits at C2/3 and is grasped with forceps. The T-saw is then passed through the tube, and each end of the saw is clamped. The T-saw runs in the epidural space from C3 to C7. While working the T-saw, care must be taken not to pull up on the saw and cause cervical kyphosis. We have developed a device that helps to maintain lordosis during sawing (Fig. 2).

The saw should be irrigated with sterile saline to minimize friction and heat. It is also important to ensure that the T-saw is centered in the midline of each spinous process. Midline splitting is achieved within a few minutes, but if it is difficult to insert the epidural tube, such as in cases of severe stenosis, the narrowest interlaminal space should be opened carefully using the same procedure as for C7/Th1. Then midline splitting should be carried out

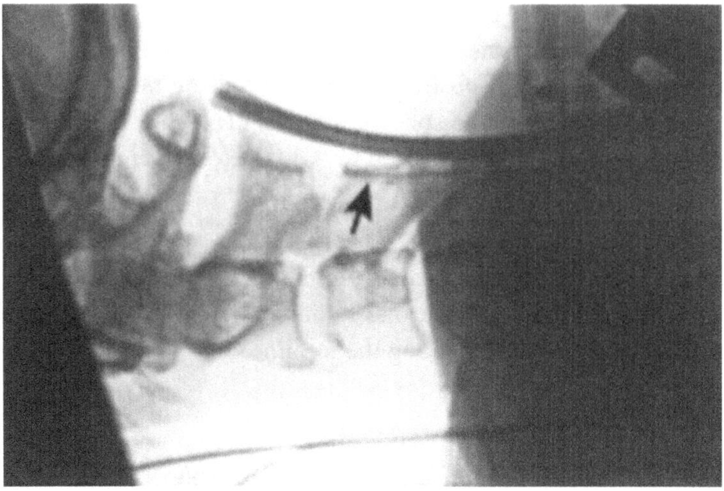

Fig. 2. Intraoperative imaging. There is no risk of damage to the spinal cord if cervical lordosis is maintained during the splitting of the spinous processes. The *arrow* indicates the T-saw

separately. If a T-saw is not available, a small Kerrison rongeur is recommended to split the remaining spinous processes one by one to make a bilateral gutter.

Making a Bilateral Hinge

The line of the lateral gutter is located at the transitional area between the lamina and the articular process. Using an air-drill with a 3-mm round diamond bur, the outer cortex is cut and thinned. Each lamina is opened bilaterally from the cephalad to the caudal direction using Metsenbaum scissors and a 3-0 curette. If the lamina is difficult to open, it should be thinned further until it is more elastic. Opening the lamina of C7 is achieved after cutting the yellow ligament of C7/Th1.

Confirmation of Decompression

Adhesion between the dura and the yellow ligament is carefully stripped with a small elevator. If possible, posterior translation and good pulsation of the spinal cord should be confirmed by intraoperative ultrasound sonography.

Stabilization of the HA Spacer (Fig. 3)

A test should be carried out to determine the width of the spacer needed. The test spacers have small flanges to prevent displacement. A 15-mm spacer

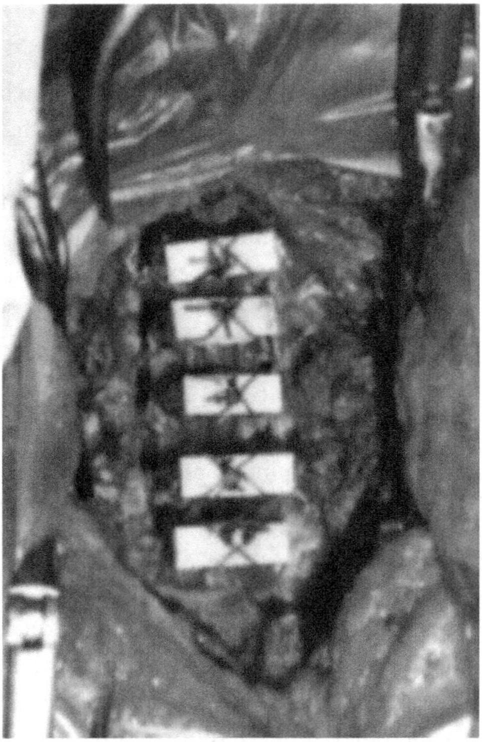

Fig. 3. The stabilization of hydroxyapatite spacers from C3 to C7

is usually used at C3 or C4, and a 20-mm spacer at lower levels. A diamond bur 2 mm in diameter is used to make holes for the sutures which tie each spacer to the lateral walls of the spinous process. A spacer is tightly fixed between the sides of the split lamina with two nonabsorbable thread sutures. We use an instant glue (Alon-alfa, Sankyo, Tokyo, Japan) to prevent loosening of the knots. In the elderly and those with osteoporotic bone, care must be taken not to collapse the laminae at the lateral gutter while tying the sutures. In cases of cervical instability, an autogenous iliac bone graft is used for the unstable segment instead of a HA spacer, and bone chips are placed on the bilateral gutters.

Reattachment of the Semispinal Muscle and Closure

The cervical semispinal muscles are reattached to the spinous process of C2. This helps to prevent postoperative kyphotic change, which is a poor prognostic factor following laminoplasty. If the spinous process is too weak to anchor the muscles, the contralateral rectus capitus muscles are used to tie them. A suction drainage tube is placed on the laminae, and the wound is closed by layer.

Postoperative Care

The suction drainage tube is removed within 24h. Two days after the operation, sitting and walking are permitted with a Philadelphia collar. Two weeks postoperatively, isometric exercises of the neck and shoulder girdle are started, and a soft collar can replace the Philadelphia collar. Early muscle exercises are recommended to maintain the range of motion (ROM) of the neck. Four weeks postoperatively, the soft collar can be removed.

Complications of this Laminoplasty Procedure

Maladaptation of the HA Spacer to the Split Spinous Process

The tip of the spinous process must be cut very precisely to accommodate a spacer between the split ends of the lamina.

C5 Nerve Palsy

In the first few days after the operation, pain may occur in the shoulder or the upper arm. Later, weakness of the deltoid and the biceps brachii muscles may develop. This palsy is usually motor dominant. It has been suggested that a tethered nerve root resulting from posterior translation of the spinal cord, could be a major cause (see the chapter by N. Tsuzuki in this volume). Nonsteroidal antiinflammatory drugs and neck rest, e.g., neck traction in the neutral position, should relieve the pain, and the muscle weakness should gradually resolve within 12 months.

Pitfalls of this Procedure

Some of the problems associated with our procedure are:

1. Making the lateral gutter too near the outer edge may cause facet fusion.
2. Using the T-saw in the flexion position may damage the spinal cord. Maintaining lordosis is important.
3. In cases with fragile bones, pulling the suture thread too tight while stabilizing the HA spacer may destroy the lateral gutter.

Radiographic Results

To evaluate the results of our method radiographically, we compared a group using HA spacers with a group using iliac bone grafts. Lateral radiographs taken in the neutral, flexion, and extension positions before surgery and

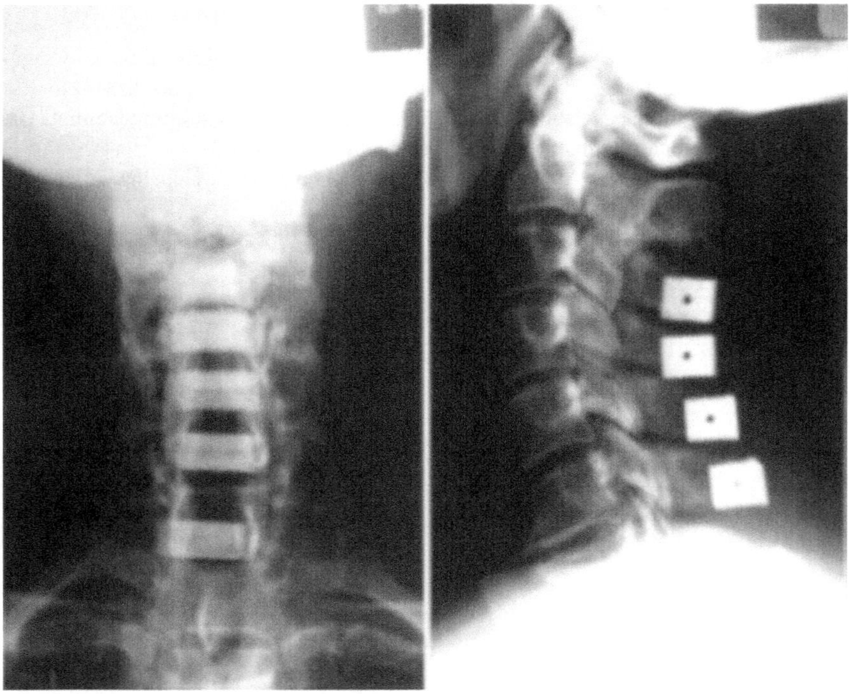

Fig. 4. Lateral radiographs showing a good alignment 6 months postoperatively

again at the final follow-up were used to measure the ROM at C2–7. The ROM of the group with HA spacers (mean follow-up 25.0 months, $n = 49$ cases) was $37° \pm 15°$ preoperatively and $19° \pm 12°$ at final follow-up. The ROM of the group with autogenous iliac bone grafts (mean follow-up 62.4 months, $n = 15$ cases) was $42° \pm 15°$ preoperatively and $8.9° \pm 10°$ at final follow-up. The ROM of the occipital–C1 and C1–2 tends to increase at the expense of the ROM of C2–7. HA spacers effectively maintain the ROM of the cervical spine (Fig. 4).

This method of laminoplasty has several advantages:

1. shorter operating times using HA spacers and a T-saw;
2. full expansion of the spinal canal;
3. prevention of postoperative kyphotic change;
4. maintenance of the ROM of the cervical spine;
5. decompression of the nerve root by partial facetectomy; and
6. prevention of spinal instability by using a bone block instead of a HA spacer, or by placing bone chips on the bilateral gutters.

References

1. Kurokawa T, Tsuyama N, Tanaka H, et al. (1982) Enlargement of spinal canal by sagittal splitting of the spinous process (in Japanese). Bessatsu Seikeigeka 2:234–240
2. Nakano K, Harata S, Suetsuna F, et al. (1992) Spinous process-splitting laminoplasty using hydroxyapatite spinous process spacer. Spine 17:S41–S43
3. Yonenobu K, Yamamoto T, Ono K (1998) Laminoplasty for myelopathy. Lippincott-Raven, Philadelphia, pp 849–864

Bilateral Open Laminoplasty Using the Spinous Process as Bone Blocks

Ikuo Aita[1], Takeshi Yabuki[2], and Yasuyoshi Wadano[3]

Introduction

Laminoplasty consists of enlargement of the spinal canal and reconstruction of the lamina. There are two basic methods for enlargement of the spinal canal. One involves splitting the center of the lamina and opening the lamina bilaterally, the so-called French door approach [1]. The other method, known as Hirabayashi's open door [2], involves cutting the lateral side of the lamina and then opening the lamina to the other side.

Reconstruction of the lamina is performed with a spacer, usually hydroxyapatite (HA) [3], iliac bone, or part of the spinous process. The lateral gutter, where the lamina is thinned sufficiently to be turned posteriorly, gradually becomes thick and strong after the operation [4]. Therefore, reconstruction of the lamina with a bone spacer is not absolutely necessary, although, we think that it is preferable. There has been a report of shortening of the spinous process in patients with HA spacers [5], which is another reason for recommending the use of bone spacers.

We use a French door-type laminoplasty, with spacers made from the spinous processes. Before splitting the center of the lamina, we cut the spinous process at the base. Thereafter, splitting the center of the lamina is easy and safe, and harvesting bone blocks from the iliac crest is unnecessary. Bone union is good in our procedure.

[1] Department of Orthopaedic Surgery, Institute of Clinical Medicine, University of Tsukuba, Tennohdai 1-1-1, Tsukuba, Ibaraki 305-8575, Japan
[2] Yabuki Orthopaedic Clinic, 2-12-18 Keyakidai, Moriya, Ibaraki 302-0128, Japan
[3] Department of Orthopaedics, Center for Medical Sciences, Ibaraki Prefectural University of Health Science, 4669-2 Ami-machi, Inashiki-gun, Ibaraki 300-0394, Japan

Indications

The indications for this type of surgery are definite neurological impairment and evidence of spinal cord compression on radiological imaging. Patients with symptoms of motor dysfunction should undergo the surgery to prevent severe functional disability, as myelopathy causes irreversible damage. For patients who have only sensory disturbance and no motor dysfunction, we impose immobilization with a collar. If there is little response to the neck collar or if the symptoms worsen, we consider surgery to be necessary.

Good indications for laminoplasty are a developmentally narrow canal and continuous-type or combined-type ossification of the posterior longitudinal ligament. If the spinal cord compression is mainly on the anterior side and within two segments without severe developmental canal stenosis, anterior decompression is indicated.

Operative Procedures

A skin incision is made from the inferior margin of the occipital bone to the spinous process of the first thoracic vertebra. After dissection of subcutaneous fatty tissue, the ligamentum nuchae is split longitudinally. Care should be taken not to damage the muscles. Then the insertion of paravertebral muscle into the spinous process is resected from C3 to C7. Insertion of the semispinalis cervicis muscles to the spinous process of the axis is preserved to maintain the lordotic curvature of the cervical spine. The paravertebral muscles are elevated subperiosteally, and the posterior surface of the lamina is exposed.

The spinous processes are removed at the base (Fig. 1). The narrowest sites of the spinous processes are cut at C3, C4, and C5. However, care should be taken not to cut the spinous processes too much, or the reconstruction of the lamina may be problematic because the spacer will be difficult to fix between the opened laminae. The spinous processes of C6 and C7 are longer and can be cut more than those of C3, C4, and C5.

The center of each lamina is thinned using a high-speed drill with a 2.0-mm diameter diamond burr (Fig. 2). Cancellous bone can then be removed without difficulty. Thin the ventral cortex very carefully and divide the lamina by cracking with a blunt raspatory (Fig. 2). If the ventral cortex is thin enough to crack, the caudal portion of the inner cortex looks yellow and the cephalic portion looks red because of the yellow ligament and the epidural veins, respectively. As the spinous process has already been cut, these procedures can be directly visualized and undertaken safely.

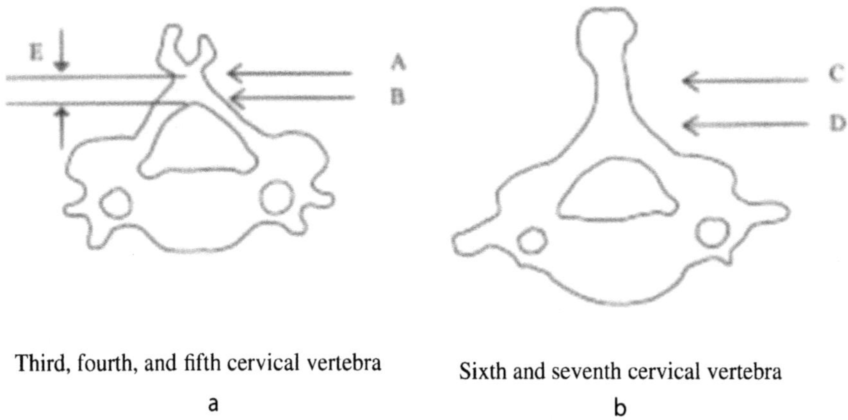

Fig. 1. Illustrations of the cut levels of the spinous processes. In C3, C4, and C5 (**a**), the spinous process is short. Cut line *A* is appropriate; cut line *B* is too deep and dangerous. In C6 and C7 (**b**), cut line *D* is appropriate. If the residual process is too long, the result of cutting at line *C* and then cutting the center of the lamina becomes more problematic as the tip of the drill bur is difficult to see. The distance between the cut level and the posterior margin of the spinal canal (*E*) should be about 5 mm for the fixation of bone blocks

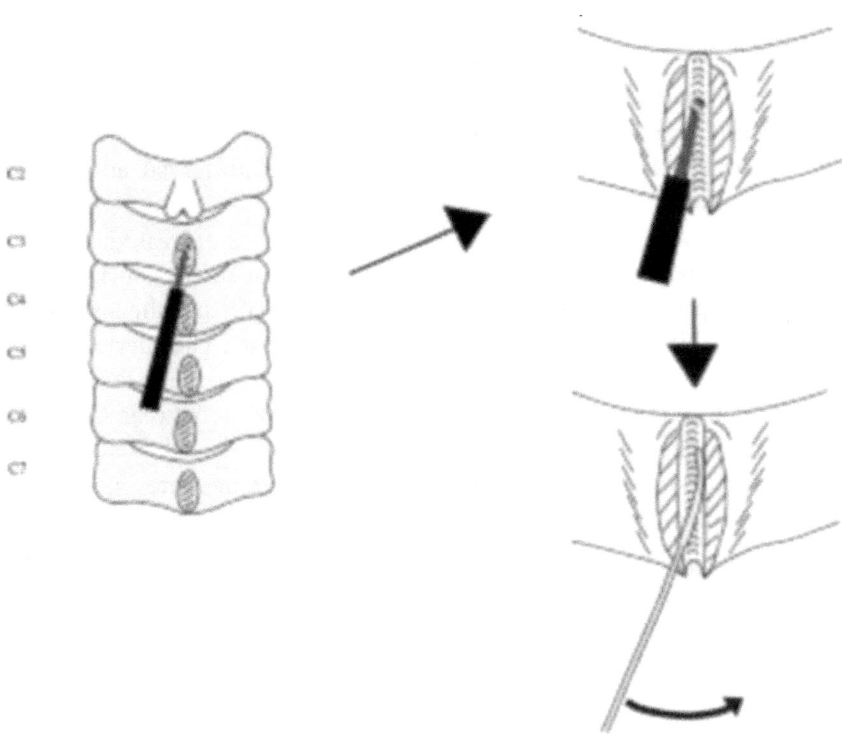

Fig. 2. The center of the lamina is thinned with a high-speed drill bur and can be directly visualized. We normally use a diamond bur 2 mm in diameter. We then crack the center of the lamina with a blunt raspatory. Using this procedure, injury to the spinal cord and the dura mater is avoided

A lateral gutter is made at the transitional portion of the lamina and the facet joint with a diamond burr 4.0 mm in diameter. The position of the lateral gutter must be checked carefully on computed tomographic myelography before the operation. Usually, the transitional portion of the lamina and the facet joint is easily identified at C5. Deepen the gutter until the ventral cortex of the lamina is exposed, but do not cut out all of the lamina. Exposure of the proximal portion of the C3 lamina is slightly difficult, because the insertion of the semispinalis cervicis muscle into the spinous process of the axis is preserved to maintain the lordotic curvature of the cervical spine. We retract the superior muscles and make a lateral gutter first at one side, and then at the other.

Elect the lamina with a bone curette. If the hinge site is too strong, drill the ventral cortex of the gutter further. However, care must be taken not to drill the gutter too much. If the ventral cortex of the lateral gutter becomes too weak, the stability of the reconstructed lamina may decrease.

The center of the ligamentum flavum is cut with scissors or a knife, and then the laminae are opened. After opening the laminae, the intersurface between the dura mater and the lamina is released. However, there is seldom any adhesion between the laminae and the dura.

After these procedures, the dura mater becomes swollen and shows good pulsation. Constricting fibrous tissues are sometimes present and need to be resected, but the extradural veins should be preserved as much as possible.

If there is a stenosis, or if the subarachnoid space is decreased at C2–3, a domed-type laminotomy of the C2 is performed. The inferior surface of the C2 spinous process is carefully exposed so as not to disturb the insertion of the semispinalis cervicis muscle more than is necessary. The inferior portion of the C2 lamina should then be removed with a high-speed drill bar. We always remove the lamina until the ligamentum flavum between C2 and C3 is free from C2.

Bone blocks to fix between the opened laminae are made from the resected spinous processes (Fig. 3). Two holes are made at the edges of the opened laminae using a small cutting bur. A bone block made from a spinous process is then fixed as shown in Fig. 4. If the bone block is wide and there is a possibility that it may collide with adjacent blocks when the cervical spine is in the extension position, the width should be decreased.

The important point is that the bilateral muscles must be drawn closely together and the ligamentum nuchae must be sutured tightly. We know that these muscles are important dynamic stabilizers for maintaining lordosis of the cervical spine, and care must be taken not to damage them, and to perform as much anatomical repair as possible.

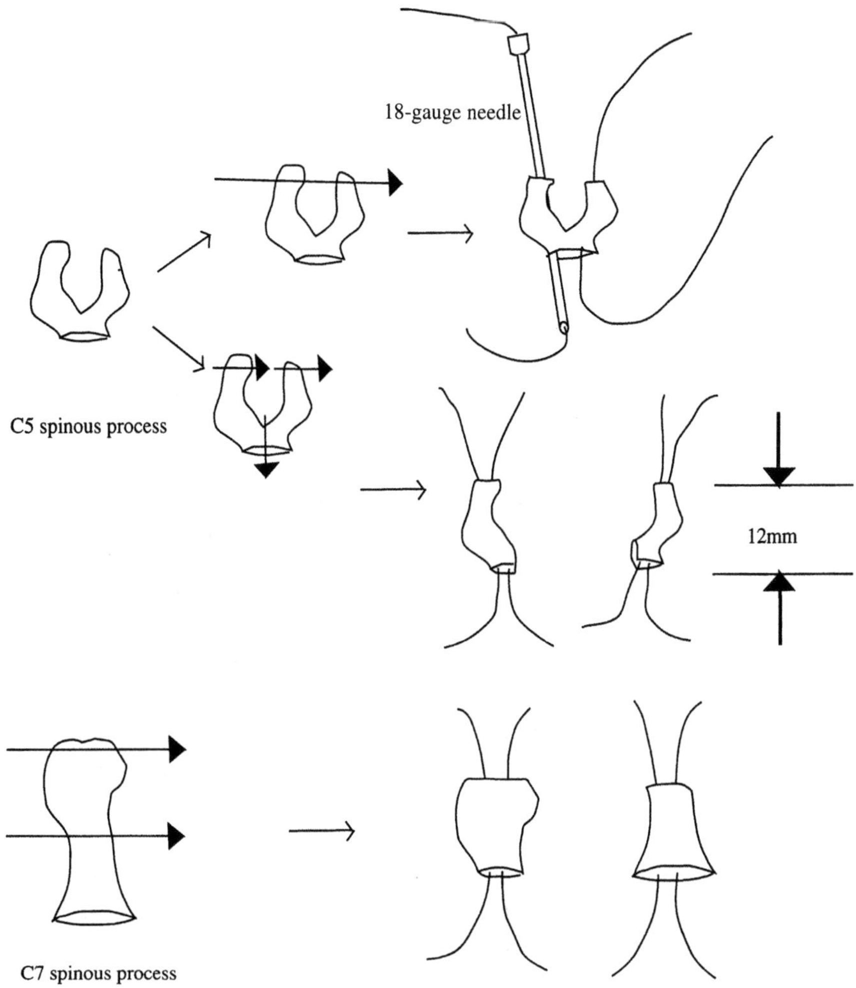

Fig. 3. Illustration of how to make a bone block from the spinous processes. The tip of the spinous process is resected and two nonabsorbable sutures are passed through the bone block with an 18-gauge needle. If the spinous process of C5 is large, two bone blocks can be made. Similarly, we can also make two bone blocks from the spinous process of C7. We think that the appropriate length of a bone block is about 12 mm

Clinical results

Thirty-five patients (26 men and 7 women) who underwent laminoplasty were followed clinically for more than 5 years and the results were analyzed. Their ages ranged from 30 to 85 years (mean 56 years) at the time of surgery. Seventeen had cervical spondylotic myelopathy and 16 had ossification of the posterior longitudinal ligament (OPLL). The remaining two cases had

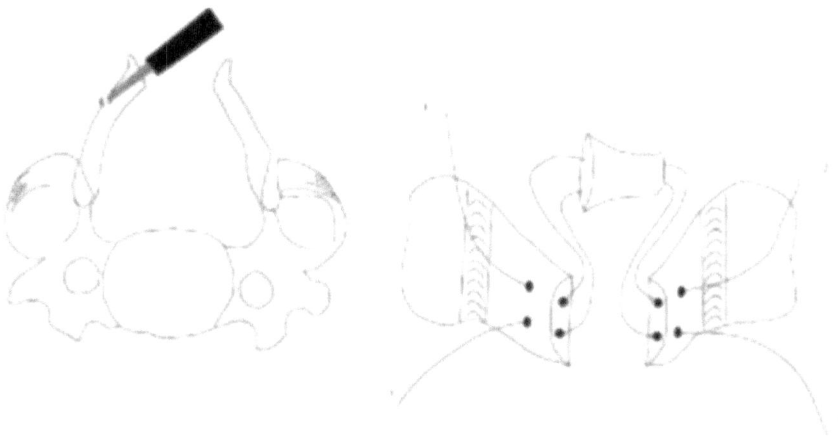

Fig. 4. Two holes are made on each side at the edge of the lamina with a high-speed drill bur. The bone blocks are then fixed with two nonabsorbable sutures. Ends *1* and *2* are tied first, then ends *3* and *4*. Then all four ends are tied together

hypertrophy of the posterior longitudinal ligament and calcification of the ligamentum flavum. The follow-up period was from 5 to 10 years (mean 7 years and 2 months). However, these patients differed in one procedure. In some cases, we temporarily dissected the insertion of the semispinalis cervicis muscle to the C2 spinous process and then repaired it before closing the wound. Most of the surgeries involved from C3 to C7 only.

Using the Japanese Orthopaedic Association scale for cervical spondylotic myelopathy, the mean preoperative score was 10.0 ± 2.9, and the mean postoperative score was 12.1 ± 2.8. The mean recovery rate [6] was 25.8% ± 40.0%.

By radiological analysis, the preoperative angle of C2–6 was 17.9° ± 13.4° and the postoperative angle was 10.1° ± 12.8°. The mean rate of decrease was 56.4%. There were two cases of increased kyphosis, and one case of curvature change to a sigmoid shape. These curvature changes were not associated with clinical deterioration. The range of motion decreased after surgery from 39.7 ± 13.2 to 13.2 ± 10.8. The mean rate of decrease was 33.2%.

Discussion

The spinal decompression effect of laminoplasty is based on posterior decompression, and the curvature of the cervical spine influences the degree of decompression. If the patient has anterior localized cord compression or local kyphosis, posterior decompression by laminoplasty may decrease the decompressive effect. After laminoplasty, the curvature of the cervical spine decreases the lordosis, and therefore an effort must be made to maintain lordosis to the extent possible. We do not resect the insertion of the semispinalis cervicis muscle to the spinous process of the axis during the operation, and we draw the bilateral muscles closely together and suture the ligamentum nuchae tightly.

Before splitting the center of the lamina, we cut the spinous process at its base. Therefore, splitting the center of the lamina is easy and safe. Moreover, there is no need to harvest bone blocks from the iliac crest. The stability of the bone block is satisfactory, and in our experience a bone block made from the spinous process is much more stable than a HA spacer. Bone blocks made from spinous process are usually long enough to enlarge the spinal canal [7].

There is a question about the reattachment of the paravertebral muscle to the spinous process. If the muscles reattach to the spinous process, it is better to preserve the spinous process. However, we have no data on this point.

The stability of the cervical spine after this type of laminoplasty is good, and we have gradually speeded up the postsurgical rehabilitation. In our early trials, patients were allowed to sit and walk 2 weeks after surgery. Now, however, they are permitted to do so 1 week postsurgery. The period of wearing a neck orthosis is 4 weeks. We think that providing a physiological load to the cervical spine soon after the operation has a positive effect on its curvature, and an even earlier program of rehabilitation may be possible.

References

1. Kurokawa T, Tanaka H, Kobayashi M, et al. (1982) Enlargement of the spinal canal by the sagittal splitting of the spinous process. Bessatsu Seikeigeka 2:234–240
2. Hirabayashi K, Watanabe K, Wakano K, et al. (1983) Expansive open-door laminoplasty for cervical spinal stenotic myelopathy. Spine 8:693–699
3. Nakano K, Harata S, Suetsuna F, et al. (1992) Spinous process-splitting laminoplasty using hydroxyapatite spinous process spacer. Spine 17:S41–S43
4. Hirabayashi K, Satomi K (1988) Operative procedure and results of expansive open-door laminoplasty. Spine 13:870–876
5. Hoshi K, Kurokawa T, Nakamura K, et al. (1996) Expansive cervical laminoplasties. Observations on comparative changes in spinous process lengths following longitudinal laminal division using autogenous bone or hydroxyapatite spacers. Spinal Cord 34:725–728
6. Hase H, Watanabe T, Hirasawa, et al. (1991) Bilateral open laminoplasty using ceramic laminas for cervical myelopathy. Spine 16:1269–1276
7. Aita I, HayAshi K, Wadano Y, et al. (1998) Posterior movement and enlargement of the spinal cord after cervical laminoplasty. J Bone Joint Surg 80:33–37

Expansive Midline T-Saw (Modified Spinous Process-Splitting) Laminoplasty for the Treatment of Cervical Myelopathy

Norio Kawahara, Katsuro Tomita, Tadayoshi Kobayashi, Hideki Murakami, Tomoyuki Akamaru, and Koshi Nanbu

Introduction

Laminoplasty procedures for cervical myelopathy were evolved in Japan [1–5]. Open-door laminoplasty was introduced by Hirabayashi in 1978 [1]. Many variations have been described, including sagittal splitting of the spinous processes described Kurokawa et al. in 1982 [4]. In this procedure, spinal canal enlargement is achieved by sagittal splitting of the spinous process with a bur. After opening the hinged hemilaminae to the sides, several blocks of autograft bone are inserted between the two halves and stabilized with wire [4]. This procedure has a number of theoretical and practical advantages. First, the posterior arch can be reconstructed symmetrically as each hemilamina opens on its own hinge. Second, the enlargement of the spinal canal is constantly maintained by the bone grafts [4]. Third, troublesome hemorrhage from the arborizing lateral epidural veins is avoided since there are few veins in the dorsal midline epidural space. To date, the principal disadvantage of the midline spinous process splitting techniques has been the technical difficulty because of the high risk of cord injury during sagittal splitting with a bur. We have developed a safe sagittal splitting technique using a threadwire saw (T-saw, Fig. 1) [6] and called "expansive midline T-saw laminoplasty" [7].

Department of Orthopaedic Surgery, School of Medicine, Kanazawa University, 13-1 Takara-machi, Kanazawa 920-8641, Japan

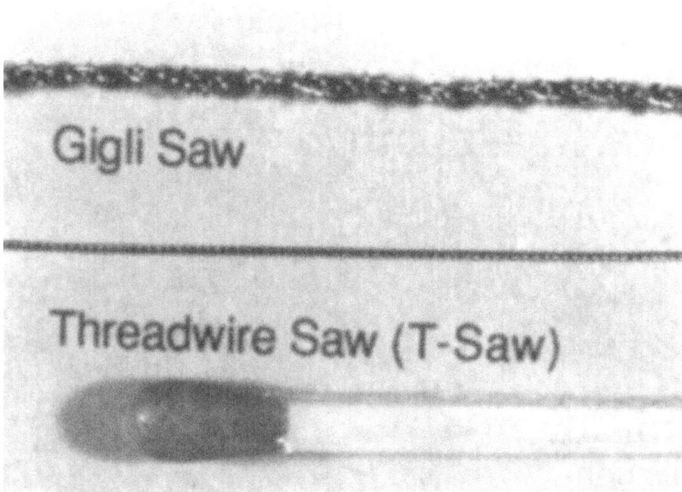

Fig. 1. A Gigli saw, a threadwire saw (T-saw), and a match

Materials and Methods

Surgical Technique

Position and Exposure

The patient is intubated, with all necessary precautions taken in case pathologic spinal cord compression is present. The positioning and preparation of the operative field proceed as for any multilevel posterior cervical exposure. The neck should not be positioned in kyphosis. Preoperative determination of the patient's range of motion without symptom exacerbation helps to indicate a reasonable intraoperative alignment. A lateral X-ray should be taken to assist the cervical intraoperative aligment. A midline posterior exposure is performed, taking care to avoid detachment of the semispinalis muscles into the spinous process of C2. This maintains effective cervical extensor power, and helps to maintain cervical alignment. The paraspinal muscles are dissected, leaving the supra- and interspinous ligaments intact. Subperiosteal exposure of the posterior elements is performed to the medial portion of the lateral mass so that bone troughs can be made in the medial one-third of the lateral mass. Undue injury to the facet capsules should be avoided.

Splitting the Spinous Processes

A flavectomy in the middle portion is used to expose the midline epidural space above and below the intended levels of decompression. In most cases

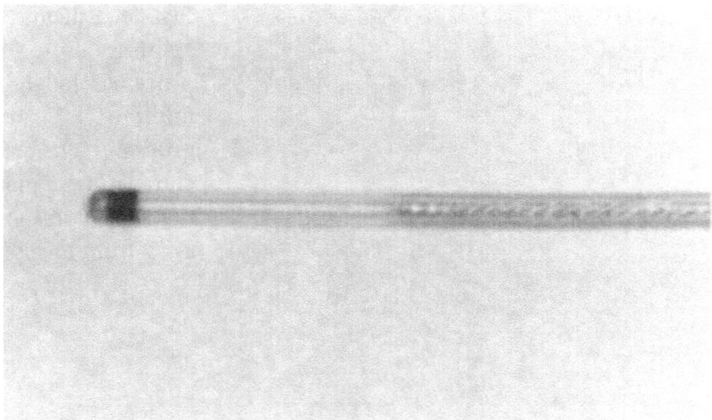

Fig. 2. The top end of a polyethylene outer sleeve with a T-saw inside

this is done at C2–3 and C7–T1, or at least one full lamina above and below the extent of the cord compression. A T-saw 0.54 mm in diameter, contained within its specially designed removable polyethylene outer sleeve (1.2 mm in diameter) (Fig. 2), is then passed along the midline epidural space from the caudal to the cranial end, or vice versa. The technique is analogous to the passage of a conventional epidural catheter or electrode. The smooth tapered tip of the outer sleeve facilitates the passage of the T-saw without damage to the meninges (Fig. 2). The advancing tip of the sleeve is grasped as it appears in the laminotomy at the opposite end of the decompression zone. The T-saw is then advanced through the sleeve so that it can be held securely while the sleeve is withdrawn back over the saw. The unsheathed saw now spans the midline of the spinal canal along the area to be decompressed. Each end is grasped with a special clamp. The T-saw is pulled tight before a reciprocating motion is initiated. The T-saw should fit snugly just at the midline of the inner wall of the laminar arch. A continuous reciprocating motion will cut the spinous processes from the ventral to the dorsal side and away from the dura and the spinal cord (Fig. 3). The reciprocating motion should be gentle to avoid spinal cord trauma. The supra- and interspinous ligaments are automatically dissected at the midline. The saw should be lubricated with sterile saline solution to avoid excessive heat or friction.

Spinal Canal Enlargement

Bilateral gutters are then made with a high-speed bur (3 mm in diameter). They are positioned in the medial one-third of the lateral mass (Fig. 4). The outer cortex and cancellous bone are removed. The second cortex is then thinned carefully to the point that the "hinge" can be bent by a repetitive application of gentle force. Ideally, the hinge will open by plastic deforma-

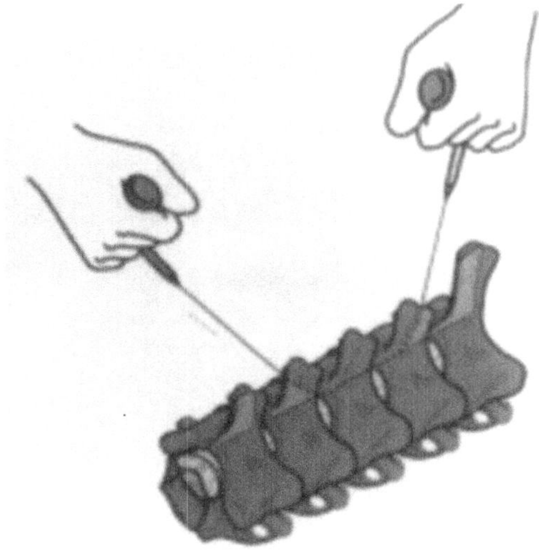

Fig. 3. Schema of midline splitting of the spinous processes by the T-saw. The midline of the spinous processes are cut with a reciprocating motion from the ventral to the dorsal side, away from the spinal cord

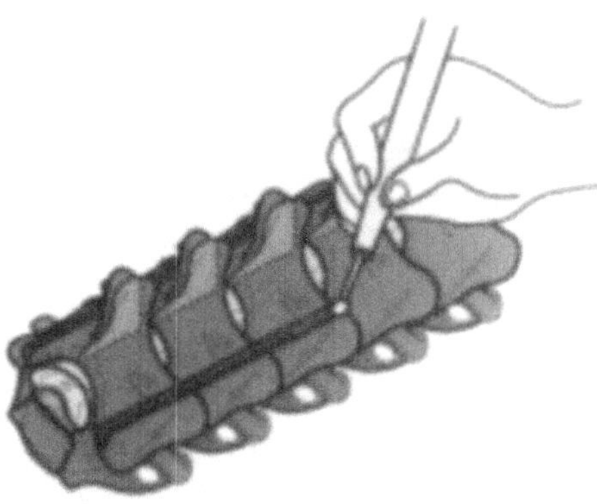

Fig. 4. Schema of the placement of gutters with a high-speed bur. Bilateral gutters are made with a high-speed bur (3 mm in diameter). They are positioned in the medial one-third of the lateral mass

tion of the bone, like a "greenstick" fracture. The split laminae are opened in sequence, like French doors, along the decompression zone, aided by the use of a modified lamina spreader (Fig. 5). Proper dural pulsation is usually observed once the hemilaminae are separated by 15–20 mm. Careful dissection of any epidural adhesions facilitates the decompression.

The decompressions typically extend from C3 through C7, but should extend one laminar level above and below the compressive pathology. If this requires additional levels caudally, the thoracic spinous processes may be split in a similar fashion. If C2 must be included, it can usually be undercut

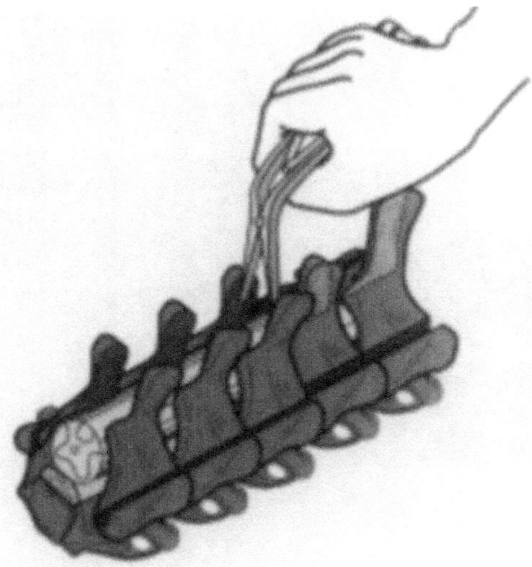

Fig. 5. Schema of the enlargement of the spinal canal. The split laminae are opened in sequence like French doors along the decompression zone, aided by the use of a modified lamina spreader

with a diamond bur without compromising its structural integrity or detaching the extensors.

Posterior Arch Reconstruction (Fig. 6)

Separation of the hemilaminae must be maintained by one of a number of techniques. If the spinous processes are well developed at C6 and C7, one can obtain as many as four hemispinous process grafts for this purpose. Corticocancellous iliac crest autografts may be employed if desired. An allograft rib or fibulae may be cut to the appropriate size and shape. Specially designed ceramic or hydroxyapatite spacers are also available for this purpose (Fig. 7). The grafts or spacers are held in place with sutures or wire passed through holes in the halves fashioned with a 1-mm bur, and/or a bone clamp.

Cautions

When the cervical canal is very narrow and the catheter cannot be passed along the entire length, or if the alignment is not lordotic, then the simultaneous cutting of all the spinous processes is contraindicated. In the case of kyphosis, the taut T-saw will be drawn like the string of a bow, possibly injuring the spinal cord by further compression (Fig. 8). In such instances, one or two additional laminotomies should be made so that only two or three levels are cut at one time (Fig. 8). In the case of scoliosis, simultaneous cut-

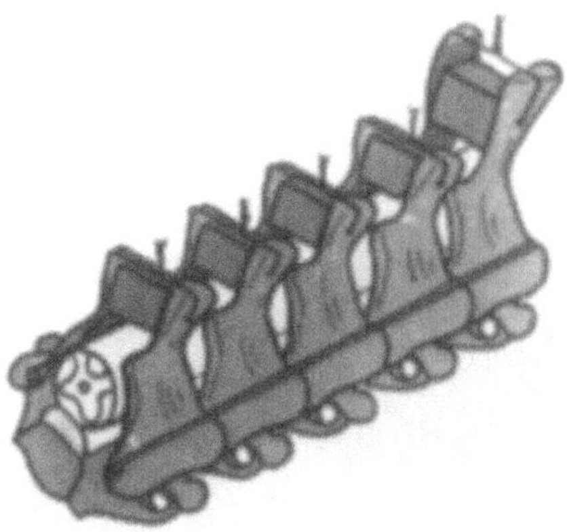

Fig. 6. Schema of the posterior arch reconstruction. Separation of the hemilaminae must be maintained by the insertion of grafts or spacers, which are held in place with sutures or by wire passed through holes in each half

ting should also be limited to two or three levels to cut along the midline of the spinous processes. The procedure is also contraindicated in the presence of OLF or an epidural scar from previous posterior cervical procedures. Passage of the polyethylene sleeve would be either unsuccessful or dangerous in such circumstances.

Patients

Eighty-eight patients underwent expansive midline T-saw laminoplasty between 1991 and 1998 for cervical myelopathy. There were 30 women and 58 men, with a mean age of 61.3 years (range 24–82 years). Twenty-two patients had ossification of the posterior longitudinal ligament (OPLL), while 66 had congenital stenosis with superimposed degenerative changes. Postoperative follow-up ranged from 24 to 106 months (mean 62 months).

Results

In 77 cases the decompression was from C3 through C7, and in the others from C3 through C6. Simultaneous midline splitting of all the spinous processes was performed in 52 patients, and two or three levels were cut at one time, followed by cutting other levels, in 36 patients. The mean operative time was 121 min (range 91–152 min). The mean operative time at our institution for previous spinous process-splitting laminoplasty procedures using a burr was 186 min (25 patients). It generally took 60–80 min to split the

a

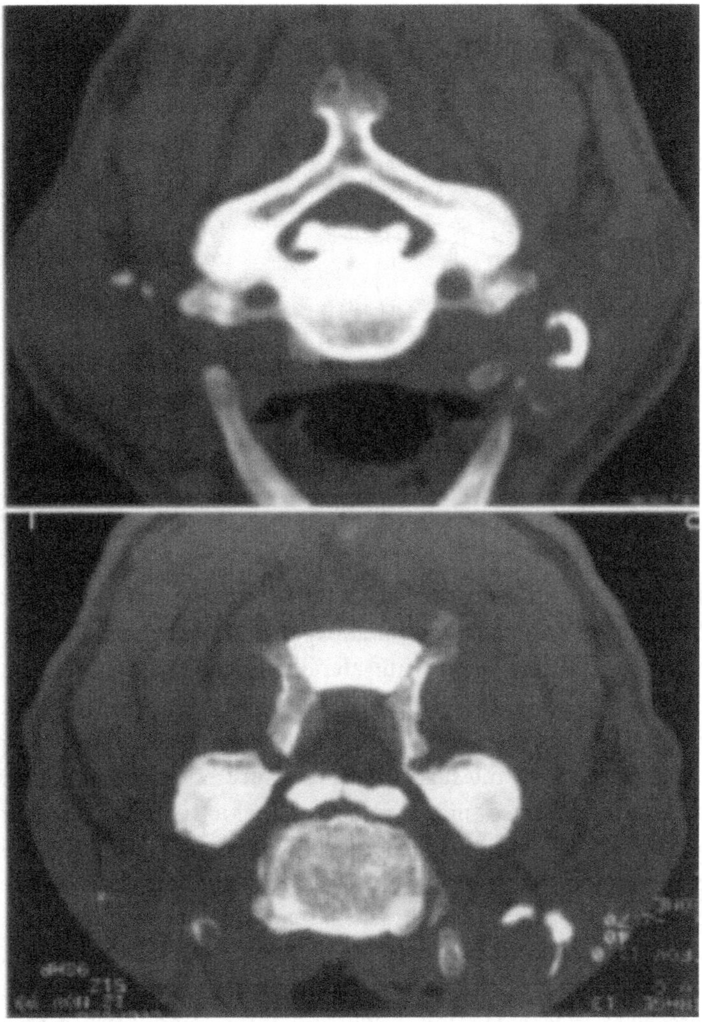

b

Fig. 7. **a** Preoperation and **b** postoperative computed tomography of the 6th cervical vertebral level of a patient with cervical myelopathy due to ossification of the posterior longitudinal ligament. Hydroxyapatite spacers were grafted between the split spinous processes

spinous process from C3 to C7 using a bur, while it took 5–10 min using the T-saw technique. Thus, the T-saw procedures were, on average, 65 min faster than the previous technique. The mean blood loss was 132 cc (range 45–320 cc), which was 70 cc less than that using a bur. No patient required a blood transfusion. No dural tears occurred, and no patient experienced any decrease in neurological function. No other complications were noted.

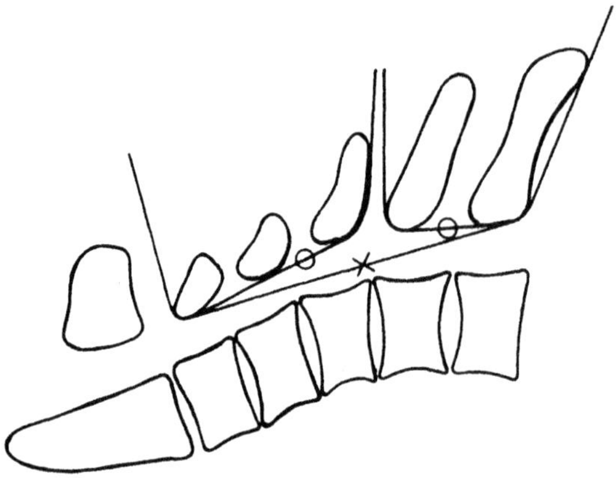

Fig. 8. Caution in cases of kyphosis. In a case of kyphosis, the taut T-saw is drawn like the string of a bow, and might injure the spinal cord by further compression. In such instances, one or two additional laminotomies should be made so that only two or three levels are cut at one time

Discussion

A spinous process-splitting laminoplasty was first described by Kurokawa et al. in 1982 [4]. The cross-sectional expansion of the spinal canal area is achieved symmetrically by creating laterally hinged hemilaminar doors that open like French doors. The original spinous process-splitting procedures employed high-speed burs with 1–3-mm bits to divide the spinous processes [4]. In such operations, the surgeon proceeds from the dorsal to the ventral side toward the meninges and the spinal cord, which entails a risk of injuring the neural tissue with the drill. Another disadvantage common to the original technique was the quantity of bone sacrificed by the bur method. The laminae were often so small or thin as to impair reconstruction of the posterior arch, especially in the midcervical levels (C3–C5). Kurokawa et al. [4] acknowledged this problem and suggested that some special device might be necessary to effect safe midline splitting of the spinous processes.

We have developed the T-saw, which is a stainless steel microcable, 0.54 mm in diameter, to perform total en bloc spondylectomy for spinal tumors [6, 8]. The T-saw has been used to facilitate the splitting of the spinous processes since 1991 [7]. This application has a number of practical advantages. The T-saw technique appears to be more time-efficient than the original technique using burrs. This time is saved during the division of the spinous processes, since the exposure, the placements of the lateral gutters, and the reconstruction are no different from those previously described. Virtually no bone is sacrificed as the spinous processes are split, which preserves more of the hemilaminae, rendering reconstruction of the new posterior arch much easier. It also permits use of the split spinous processes as local grafts in the reconstruction procedure. In addition, since the cutting proceeds from the ventral to the dorsal side, there is minimal risk to the spinal cord or dura mater, and the known risks of this procedure are reduced.

Bleeding has been less problematic because the cutting line with the T-saw is the posterior midline where the fewest epidural veins run. The cut surfaces of the spinous processes remain close together until the spinal canal enlargement. It is also effective for hemostasis.

The application of the T-saw to split the spinous processes has made Kurokawa's procedure simpler, faster, and safer.

References

1. Hirabayashi K (1978) Expansive open-door laminoplasty for cervical spondylotic myelopathy. Jpn J Surg 32:1159–1163
2. Hirabayashi K (1988) Operative procedure and results of expansive open-door laminoplasty. Spine 13:870–876
3. Hirabayashi K, Miyakawa J, Satomi K, et al. (1981) Operative results and postoperative progression of ossification among patients with cervical posterior longitudinal ligament. Spine 6:354–364
4. Kurokawa T, Tsuyama N, Tanaka H, et al. (1982) Enlargement of spinal canal by the sagittal splitting of the spinous process. Bessatsu Seikeigeka 2:234–240
5. Tomita K, Nomura S, Umeda S, et al. (1988) Cervical laminoplasty to enlarge the spinal canal in multilevel ossification of the posterior longitudinal ligament with myelopathy. Arch Orthop Trauma Surg 107:148–153
6. Tomita K, Kawahara N (1996) The threadwire saw: a new device for cutting bone. J Bone Joint Surg 78[Am]:1915–1917
7. Tomita K, Kawahara N, Toribatake Y, et al. (1998) Expansive midline T-saw laminoplasty (modified spinous process-splitting) for the management of cervical myelopathy. Spine 23:32–37
8. Tomita K, Kawahara N, Baba H, et al. (1994) Total en bloc spondylectomy for solitary spinal metastasis. Int Orthop 18:291–298

Part 5

Complications

Complications of Open-Door Laminoplasty

Morio Matsumoto, Kazuhiro Chiba, and Yoshiaki Toyama

Introduction

Open-door laminoplasty has been established as a safe and effective surgical method for decompression of the cervical spinal cord [1–3]. However, it has potential risks of several complications, some of which are specific to this method. In this chapter, the possible causes, prevention, and management of complications related to open-door laminoplasty are described.

Postoperative Hematoma

Careful attention should be paid to neurological deterioration due to postoperative hematoma that develops acutely, or sometimes subacutely, after surgery. Symptomatic hematoma is reported to be less frequent after laminoplasty than after laminectomy [4]. The prevalence rate is estimated to be 0.6% in our institution. Failures of hemostasis during surgery and postoperative drainage may be the causes of hematoma. However, even when hemostasis is secured before wound closure, hematoma can occur. Patients with hematological diseases, liver dysfunction, anticoagulant therapy, etc., are more likely to develop postoperative hematoma and therefore need to be watched more carefully after surgery.

Signs and Symptoms

Most patients demonstrate progressive quadriplegia within several hours after surgery. Pain in the upper extremities may proceed to the onset of quadriplegia. Paralysis is sometimes dominant in the open side rather than in the hinge side, possibly because the open side has more room for blood

Department of Orthopaedic Surgery, Keio University, School of Medicine, 35 Shinanomachi, Shinjuku-ku, Tokyo 160-8582, Japan

pooling. On rare occasions, paralysis develops subacutely, i.e., several days after surgery.

Diagnosis

The diagnosis of postoperative hematoma can be made based on the patients' symptoms and magnetic resonance imaging (MRI) findings (Fig. 1). MRI typically indicates a large mass compressing the spinal cord from behind. An acute hematoma has a low signal intensity on T_1-weighted images and a high signal intensity on T_2-weighted images. In the subacute stage, a hematoma presents a high signal intensity on both T_1- and T_2-weighted images owing to the oxidation of hemoglobin.

Prevention

Hemorrhagic diathesis should be scrutinized before surgery. Anticoagulants, including aspirin, warfarin, ticlopidine hydrochloride, etc., should be stopped at the appropriate time prior to surgery. Meticulous intraoperative hemostasis should be performed. Special attention should be paid to the epidural venous plexus along the cutting margin of the lamina on the open side, where bleeding is often encountered during surgery. We place several pieces of Gelfoam® on the open-side epidural space before wound closure. A suction drain should be placed over the dura mater, and the output should be monitored. If the output is very small even immediately after surgery, the drain may be clogged, and special caution against hematoma should be exercised.

Treatment

Emergent revision of the wound is mandatory to avoid irreversible neurological deterioration. After removing a hematoma, endeavors to find and coagulate active bleeders should be made. If they are not identified, hemostatic agents, including Gelfoam®, Aviten®, fibrin glue, etc., are placed on the epidural space just medial to the cutting margin of the open-side gutter, where epidural venous plexus often develops.

Postoperative Intramedullary Lesions of the Spinal Cord

Postoperative intramedullary changes of the spinal cord are sometimes observed on MRI. T_2-weighted MR images show a bright swollen spinal cord, suggesting intramedullary edema, myelomalacia, cavitation, etc. (Fig. 2), although the true pathological background of the lesion has not been confirmed. These changes shown by MRI may reflect preexsisting

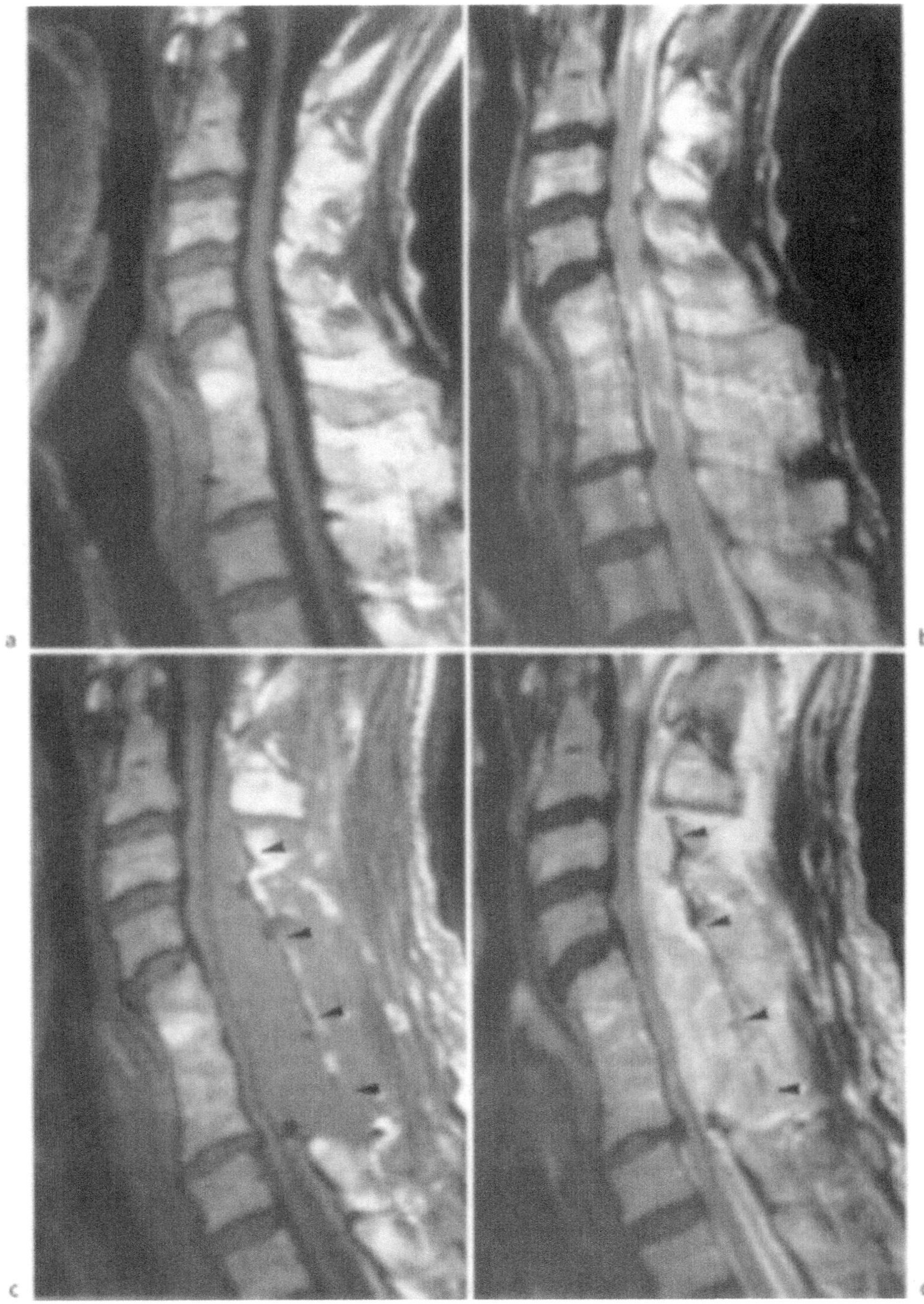

Fig. 1.

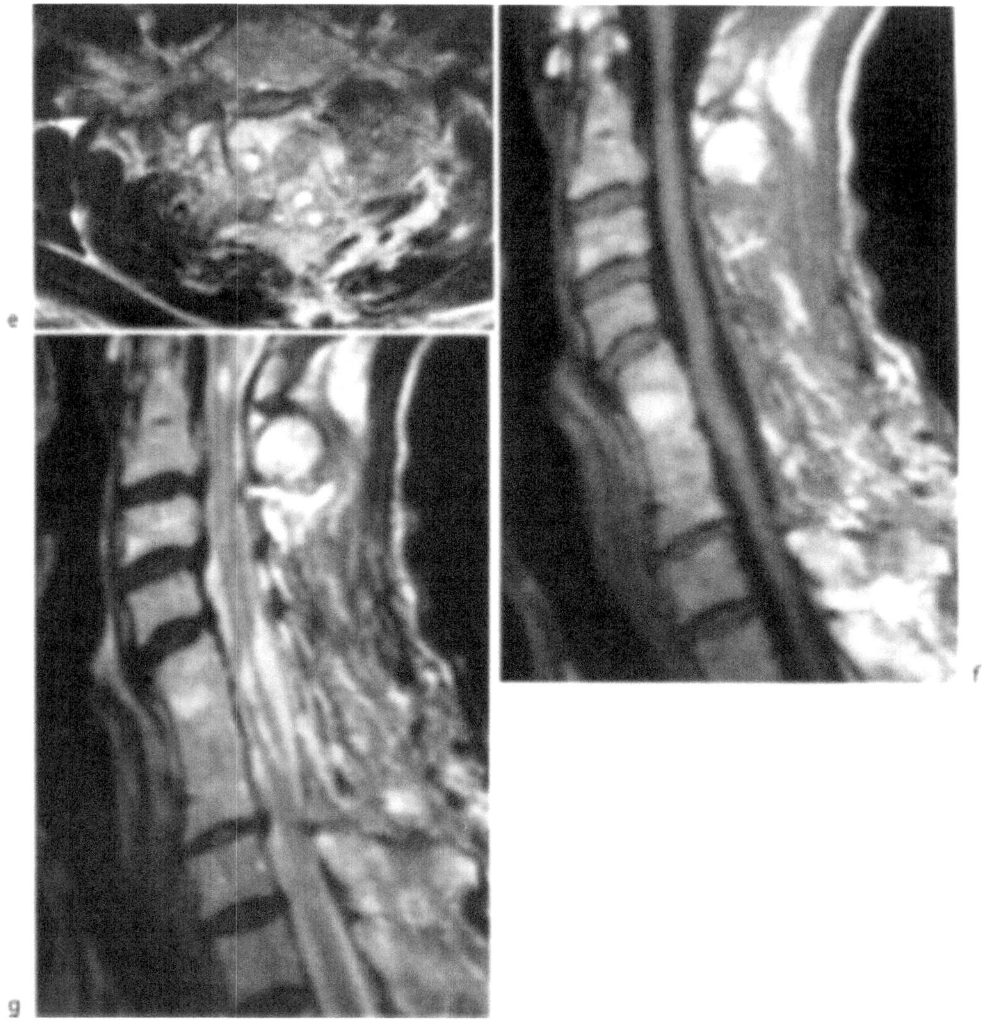

Fig. 1. A 57-year-old man underwent laminoplasty. A few hours after surgery he developed progressive quadriplegia that was more severe on the left side (open side). Magnetic resonance images (MRI) taken immediately showed that a large hematoma was compressing the spinal cord from behind. Emergency revision of the surgical wound was undertaken. The hematoma was removed, and active bleeding from the epidural vein was coagulated, followed by the placement of suction drainage. The patient recovered neurologically shortly after the revision surgery. **a, b** MRIs before surgery. **c–e** MRIs on the day of surgery. A large hematoma is compressing the spinal cord from behind (*arrowheads*). **f, g** MRIs after removal of the hamatoma

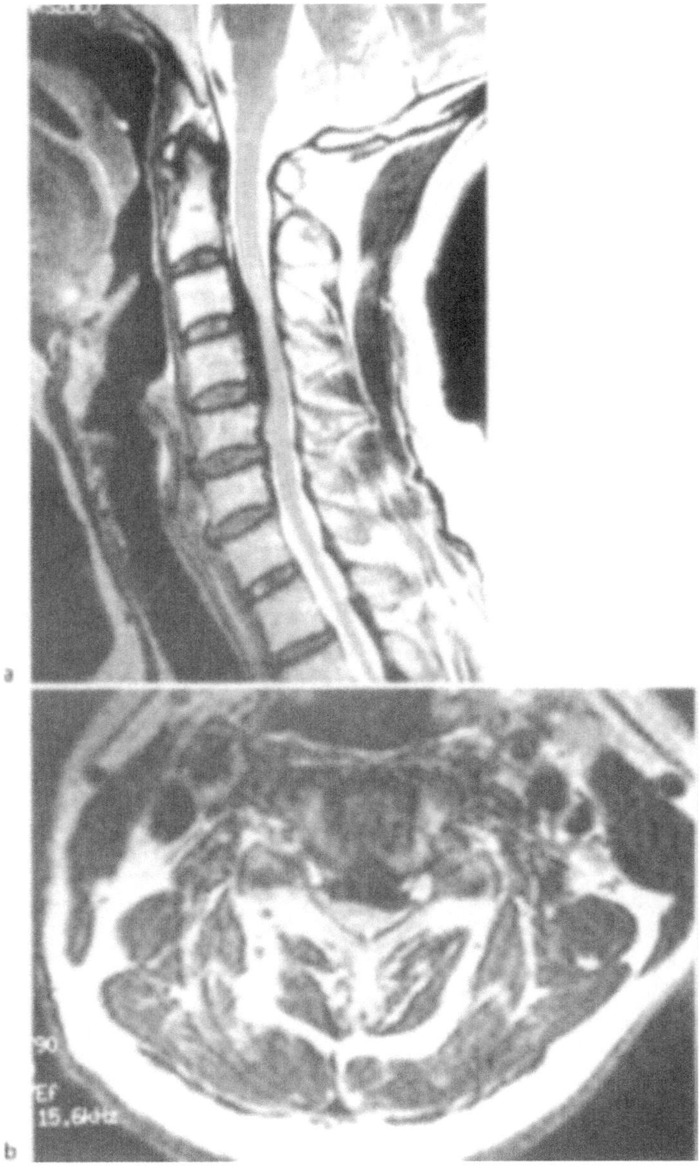

Fig. 2. A 59-year-old man with ossification of the posterior longitudinal ligament (OPLL) underwent laminoplasty with no intraoperative complications. On the day after surgery he had numbness and clumsiness in his hands which were worse than before surgery. T_2-weighted MR images showed a markedly high signal intensity area in the spinal cord extending from the C3 to the C6 level. Methylprednine was given immediately, according to the NASCIS II protocol. The patient gradually improved neurologically, but still had residual numbness and clumsiness in the hands at follow-up 1 year after surgery. **a, b** T_2-weighted sagittal images before surgery. **c, d** T_2-weighted saggital images 3 weeks after surgery. T_2-weighted axial image 3 weeks after surgery

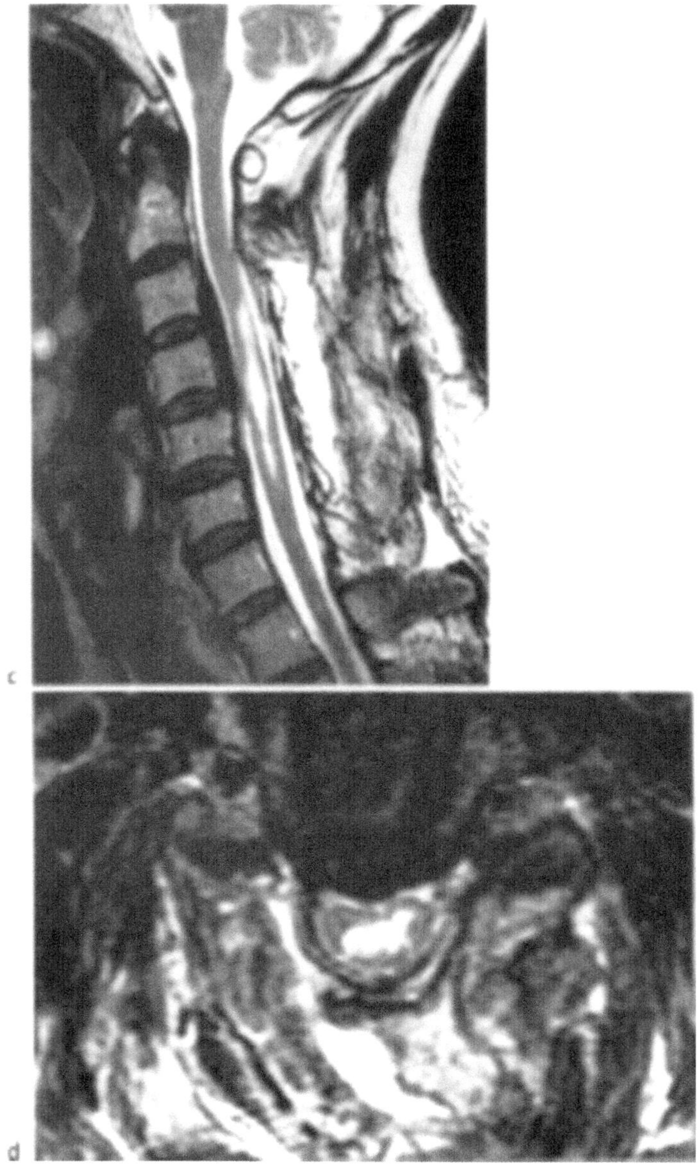

Fig. 2. *Continued*

intramedullary lesions that become notable after decompression surgery. However, on rare occasions, these changes accompany postoperative neurological deterioration shortly after surgery, even though sufficient decompression of the cervical spinal cord is achieved. In such cases, the intramedullary changes may be partly due to reperfusion of the spinal cord after decompression, as is seen in patients with cerebral embolism. This intramedullary high-signal lesion spans two or more spinal segments. Te changes of the spinal cord may last for several months, or even remain permanently.

Management and Prevention

No effective treatment has been reported for this complication. We use methylprednine according to the NASCIS II protocol immediately after the intramedullary lesion is identified on MRI in the hope that it may prevent secondary degradation of the spinal cord, although this medication has not been confirmed to be effective for this condition [5]. Also, no preventive measure has been shown to be effective.

Cerebrospinal Fluid Leaks

Cerebrospinal fluid (CSF) leaks sometimes occur during open-door laminoplasty, although their precise prevalence rate has not been determined. CSF leaks are mainly due to the laceration of the dura mater and arachnoid membrane while using the high-speed drill and Kerrison rongeur, and partly to adhesions between the dura mater and the laminae [6, 7]. CSF leaks are often not noticed until postoperative MRI or computed tomography (CT) reveals subcutaneous CSF pooling (Fig. 3).

Signs and Symptoms

CSF leaks are often asymptomatic. However, clear fluid emanating from a wound or palpation of a subcutaneous mass with fluctuation must be considered to be signs of CSF leaks. Patients sometimes complain of headache, nausea, or dizziness, which is aggravated by standing.

Prevention

Meticulous use of the high-speed drill and Kerrison rongeurs is mandatory to prevent intraoperative dural laceration. While elevating the laminae, adhesions between the dura mater and the laminae should be released gently using a Penfield dissector. When a dural tear is discovered during the procedure, it should be closed immediately.

Management

Asymptomatic CSF leaks noticed incidentally on postoperative MRI may be noted, but they will be absorbed spontaneously in most cases. However, symptomatic CSF leaks should be addressed more aggressively. Subarachnoid lumbar drainage is the most effective treatment and should be attempted first. If that fails, revision of the wound should be performed. A dural tear should be sutured or patched depending on its size. Free fat

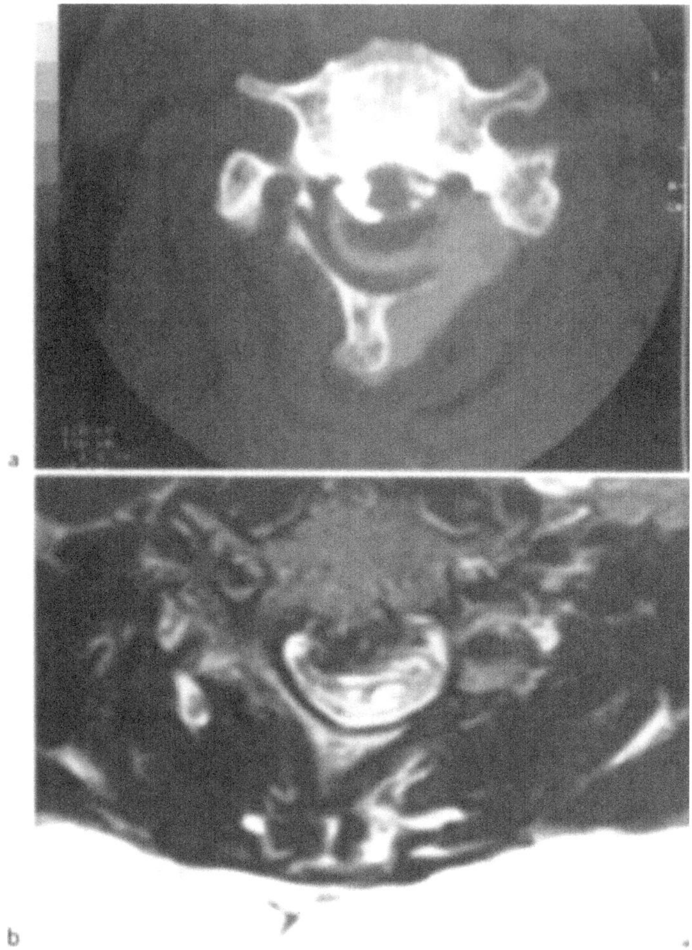

Fig. 3. A 57-year-old woman with OPLL underwent open-door laminoplasty. Although no CSF leak or dural tear was noted during surgery, she developed subcutaneous CSF pooling postoperatively with no breakdown of the surgical wound. She was followed without surgical intervention, and there was spontaneous regression of the CSF pooling. **a** Postoperative computed tomography myelogram (CTM). **b** MR image 5 years after surgery

or Gelfoam®, together with fibrin glue, are placed on the dura, and tight, layer-to-layer sutures of the muscles, subcutaneous tissues, and skin are inserted.

Lamina Fracture

The procedure of opening the laminae during laminoplasty consists of making microfractures of the laminae at the hinge. Therefore, lamina fractures are common findings on postoperative CT scans. In most cases, lamina fractures are asymptomatic, and fuse spontaneously within 1 year after surgery. However, in some cases, fractured laminae migrate into the spinal canal and compress some neural structures, resulting in root irritation and even a deterioration of the cervical myelopathy.

Signs and Symptoms

Patients with lamina fractures usually complain of pain and numbness in the upper extremities and shoulder girdle on the hinge side. Some patients have a loss of muscle strength in the upper extremities and clumsiness in the hands. These symptoms can either develop after surgery, or preoperative symptoms can become more severe after surgery. C5 palsy developing on the hinge side can sometimes be attributed to lamina fracture.

Diagnosis

CT scans show lamina fractures clearly, as well as the position of any broken lamina in the spinal canal (Fig. 4). MRI is useful to identify compression of the spinal cord and nerve roots by a migrated lamina.

Prevention

Meticulous care in drilling the laminae on the hinge side is necessary to prevent lamina fractures [1]. The gutter of the hinge should be drilled step by step, with frequent assessments of its rigidity or flexibility, until a spring-like resistance from the lamina against the lifting force is obtained. We use a diamond bur at the final stage of making the hinge so that the lamina will not become too thin. The hinges should be made slightly laterally, because hinges that are placed too medially are likely to become fractured and then compress neural structures.

Treatment

Radicular pain due to lamina fractures with mild indentation of neural structures can usually be managed conservatively by bracing and medication. Pain will often decrease within a month or two. However, for those with a deterioration of their myelopathy and marked compression of the spinal cord by a fragment of displaced lamina, immediate surgical intervention is necessary. In such cases, broken laminae need to be removed. Any attempt to reposition the laminae will result in failure.

Reclosure of the Lamina

Reclosure of laminae is a characteristic complication of open-door laminoplasty (Fig. 5). It is usually noticed on X-rays taken several days after surgery.

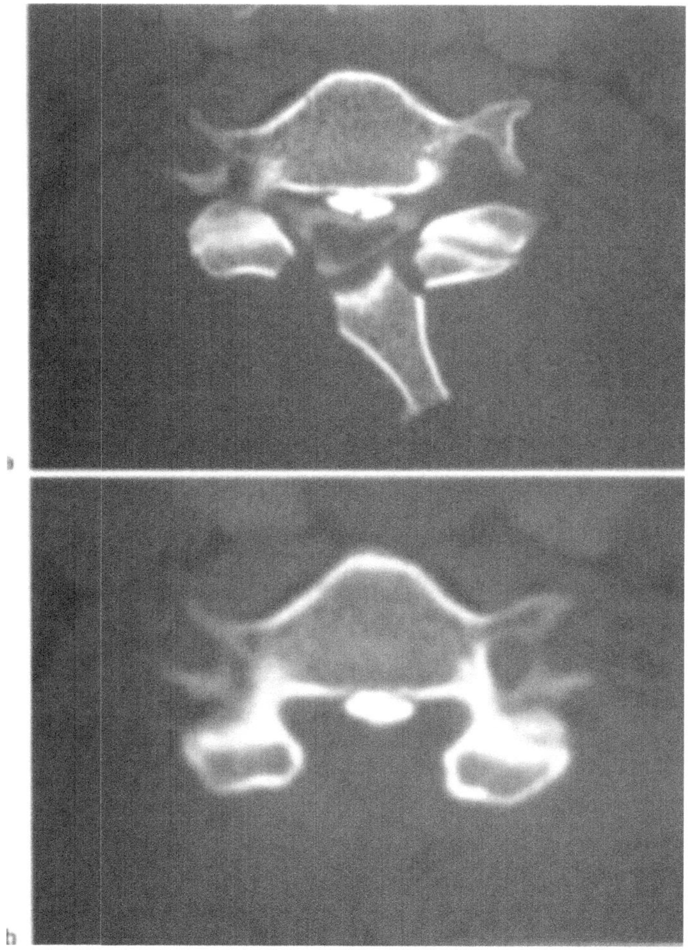

Fig. 4. A 47-year-old man with OPLL had weakness and numbness in the right upper extremity shortly after open-door laminoplasty. Postoperative computed tomography (CT) showed lamina fractures and migration of the lamina into the spinal canal. In spite of analgesics and brace treatment, there was no improvement in his symptoms, and he underwent surgical removal of the fractured lamina. **a** Postoperative CTM. Note the migrated lamina compressing the spinal cord. Also note that the gutter on the hinge side is placed slightly too medially. **b** CT after removal of the lamina

Reclosure of a lamina may be due to loosening of the retention sutures placed on the opened lamina. Reclosure of the lamina itself does not always result in recurrent neurological deterioration in the short term, because once the laminae are opened, decompression of the spinal cord can be obtained to some extent. However, in the long term, patients such as those with progressive ossification of the posterior longitudinal ligament may experience a recurrence of myelopathy.

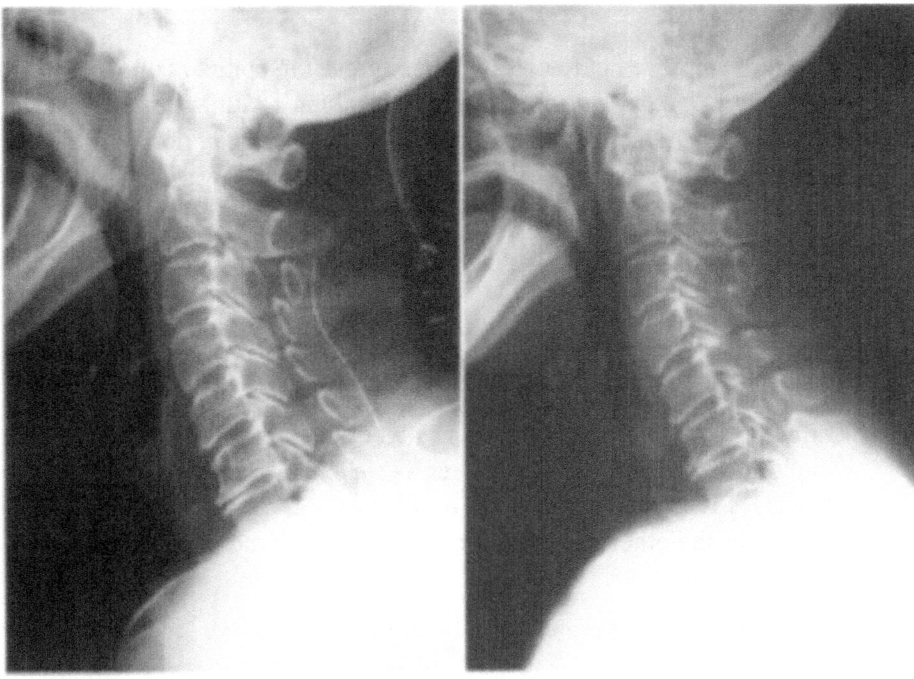

Fig. 5. A 76-year-old woman underwent open-door laminoplasty. A postoperative radiograph taken a few days after surgery showed reclosure of the laminae. Because she improved neurologically and had no recurrent symptoms during follow-up, she was observed but had no revision surgery. **a** A radiograph taken immediately after surgery. **b** A radiograph taken 2 weeks after surgery

Prevention

To avoid this complication, retention sutures should be placed as close to the facet joint on the hinge side as possible, where the multifidus muscles are tendinous and strong enough to resist any strain on these sutures [1, 2]. If a retention suture is placed close to the skin rather than to the facet joint, it may be loosened during closure of the wound at the final stage of surgery. To obtain maximum tension on the retention sutures, muscle retainers need to be loosened prior to tying the sutures, and, as Hirabayashi proposed, the cervical spine should be repositioned from flexion to a neutral position [2]. The use of bone anchors, which are placed into the lateral mass of the cervical spine, is one solution to the problem of reclosure of the laminae. A preliminary report by Wang et al. [8] indicated good outcomes with this technique. Alternative methods include the placement of bone blocks, plates, or spacers on the open side [3, 9, 10].

Management

If patients improve neurologically after surgery in spite of lamina closure, observation of their postoperative course alone is sufficient. However, if patients deteriorate neurologically during the follow-up period, or if they do not improve neurologically shortly after surgery, removal of the laminae should be considered.

Fusion of the Laminae

In patients with ossifying diathesis, such as those with ossification of the posterior longitudinal ligament, spontaneous fusion between adjacent laminae frequently occurs (Fig. 6). Fusion of the laminae may not be a true complication, since it has advantages as well as disadvantages. One of the advantages is its stabilizing effect on the cervical spine. The major disadvantage, on the other hand, is a limitation of neck movement, which frus-

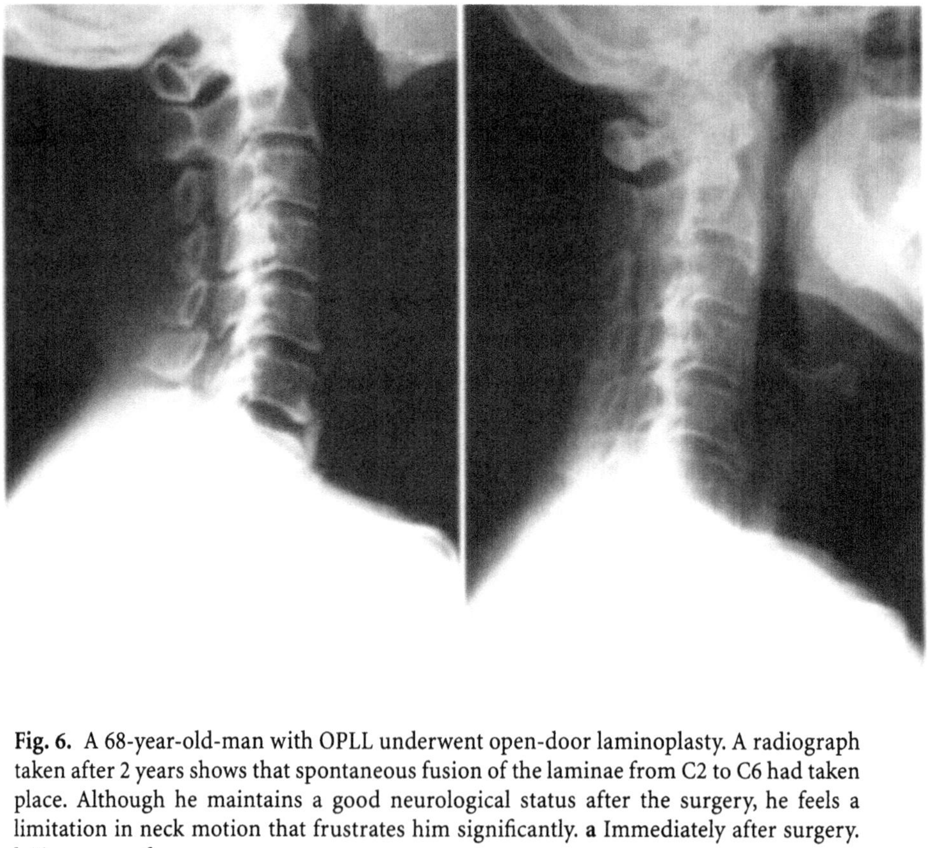

a b

Fig. 6. A 68-year-old-man with OPLL underwent open-door laminoplasty. A radiograph taken after 2 years shows that spontaneous fusion of the laminae from C2 to C6 had taken place. Although he maintains a good neurological status after the surgery, he feels a limitation in neck motion that frustrates him significantly. **a** Immediately after surgery. **b** Two years after surgery

trates many patients. To prevent this complication and also to prevent late-onset postoperative axial pain [11], prolonged postoperative bracing should be avoided, and patients should be encouraged to move the neck as early as possible after surgery. Currently, we have abandoned the routine use of a postoperative cervical brace, and we limit postoperative cervical bracing to patients whose pain is too severe for them to sit or stand upright.

Other Complications

Other complications of laminoplasty include C5 palsy, postoperative kyphosis, and postoperative axial pain. The details of these problems are discussed in the chapter by Dr. Chiba in Part 5.

References

1. Hirabayashi K, Toyama Y, Chiba K (1999) Expansive laminoplasty for myelopathy in ossification of the longitudinal ligament. Clin Orthop 359:35–48
2. Hirabayashi K, Satomi K, Toyama Y (1998) Surgical management of OPLL: anterior versus posterior approach. Part II. In: Clark CR (ed) The cervical spine, 3rd edn. Lippincott-Raven, Philadelphia, pp 876–887
3. Itoh T, Tsuji H (1985) Technical improvement and results of laminoplasty for compressive myelopathy in the cervical spine. Spine 10:729–736
4. Yonenobu K, Hosono N, Iwasaki M (1991) Neurologic complication of surgery for cervical compression myelopathy. Spine 16:1277–1282
5. Bracken MB (1993) Pharmacological treatment of acute spinal cord injury: current status and future projects. J Emerg Med 11:43–48
6. Agrillo U, Simonetti G, Martino V (1991) Postoperative CSF problems after spinal and lumbar surgery. J Neurosurg Sci 35:93–95
7. Keiper G, Stambough JL (1998) Complications of cervical spine surgery. Dural tears and cerebrospinal fluid leaks. In: Clark CR (ed) The cervical spine, 3rd edn. Lippincott-Raven, Phiadelphia, pp 899–901
8. Wang JM, Roh KJ, Kim DJ (1998) A new method of stabilizing the elevated laminae in open-door laminoplasty using an anchor system. J Bone Joint Surg 80-B:1005–1008
9. Lee TT, Manzano GR, Green BA (1997) Modified open-door cervical expansive laminoplasty for spondylotic myelopathy: operative technique, outcome, and predictors for gait improvement. J Neurosurg 86:64–68
10. O'Brien MF, Peterson D, Casey AT, et al. (1996) A novel technique for laminoplasty augmentation of the spinal canal area using titanium miniplate stabilization. A computerized morphometric analysis. Spine 21:474–483
11. Hosono N, Yonenobu K, Ono K (1996) Neck and shoulder pain after laminoplasty. A noticeable complication. Spine 21:1969–1973

Paralysis of the Arm Occurring After Decompression of the Cervical Spinal Cord

NOBUYUKI TSUZUKI, SHIGERU HIRABAYASHI, KUNIO SAIKI, and KYOKO ISHIZUKA

Postoperative Paralysis of the Arm

Paralysis of the arm has been known to occur occasionally after both posterior and anterior decompression of the cervical spinal cord without apparent mechanical trauma to the spinal cord or roots during the operation. It usually occurs as minor neurological symptoms of segmental deterioration in generally improved neurologies. Such paralysis can include both motor and sensory disturbances. The nature of the motor involvement is a lesion of the secondary motor neuron, i.e., involving the motor cell and/or anterior root, but not the long tracts of the spinal cord. This type of paralysis occurs predominantly in the C5 region and has been called C5 paralysis representatively. The primary lesions of this paralysis, i.e., whether it is of root or spinal cord origin, and the nature of the factors inducing the paralysis are not clear [1–3]. Trauma-induced paralysis, e.g., by drill penetration or laminar-edge impingement, is not discussed here.

Characteristics of the Paralysis

The following eight characteristics are common in cases of arm paralysis after spinal cord decompression.

1. It occurs after both posterior and anterior approaches.
2. It occurs even after adequate decompression without any residual bony impingement on the spinal cord or roots.
3. Three types of paralysis have been noted, i.e., a motor-dominant type, a sensory-dominant type, and a mixed type. Motor disturbance usually

Department of Orthopaedic Surgery, Saitama Medical Center, Saitama Medical School, 1981 Tsujido, Kamoda, Kawagoe, Saitama 350-8550, Japan

involves one or two motor segments with or without sensory disturbances. Sensory disturbances usually show radicular distributions. The motor-dominant type of paralysis after posterior decompression is usually accompanied by transient pain in the paralyzed area in the initial stage.
4. Pain and motor weakness can sometimes be improved by a position which reduces the nerve or root tension.
5. The paralysis is usually unilateral, and rarely bilateral.
6. The time of occurrence ranges from the first postoperative day to several months thereafter.
7. In cases with a posterior approach, the occurrence depends upon the type of laminoplasty, and ranges from 0% to 25%.
8. Except in severe cases with a manual muscle testing (MMT) score of 0 or 1, there is normally a spontaneous recovery to a useful level of movement.

Correlative Anatomy of the Dura, Spinal Cord, and Root

A root is composed of many small nerve fibers (root filaments) and can be divided into two portions, intradural and extradural. In the intradural portion, each root filament is separate and floating in the cerebrospinal fluid (CSF). In the extradural portion, the root filaments form a bundle that is covered with extensions of the dura, and this forms the sheath of the root [4] (Fig. 1). The greater part of the extradural portion of a root is located in the intervertebral foramen. In the proximal part of the foramen, the anterior root and the posterior root run independently, and in the middle of the foramen (at the pedicle level), the posterior root forms a dorsal root ganglion (DRG). Distal to the DRG, the anterior and posterior roots combine to form a spinal nerve (Fig. 2A). Proximal to the DRG, the posterior root passes through a wide portion of the intervertebral foramen, but the anterior root passes through the narrowest portion of the foramen under the superior articular process (Fig. 2B).

Changes in the Anatomical Conditions of the Dura, Spinal Cord, and Root After Decompression of the Spinal Cord

Changes in the anatomy of the dura, spinal cord, and dorsal root occur after spinal cord decompression.

1. The dural sac is enlarged by the inflow of CSF, and the compressed spinal cord expands in the CSF and moves back and forth with the pulsations

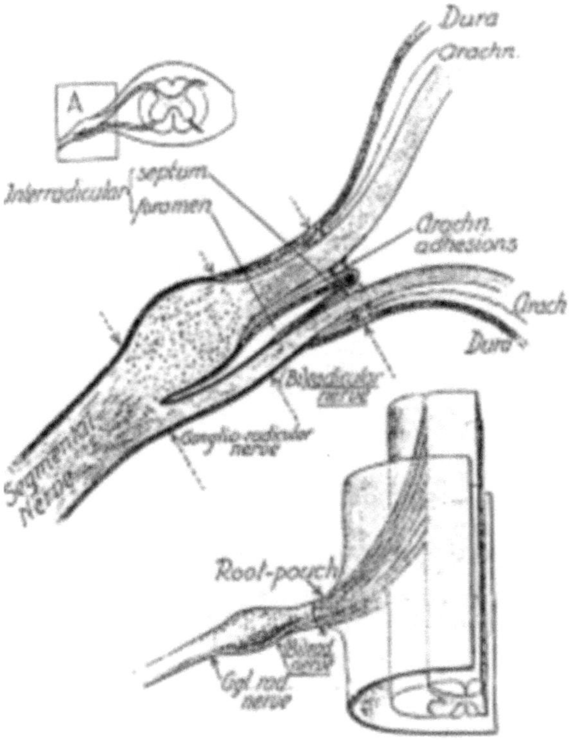

Fig. 1. Schematic representation of the correlative anatomy between the dura and the root. The radicular nerve in this drawing corresponds to the extradural portion of the root (From [4])

of the CSF. This can be confirmed by intraoperative ultrasonographic observation.

2. The tension in the root changes. The intradural portion of the root shows repeated elongation and relaxation following the pulsative movements of the spinal cord. Conversely, the extradural portion of the root becomes stretched because its neural sheath, which is an extension of the dura, is stretched by the expanded dura [5] (Fig. 3).

Possible Mechanism of Postoperative Paralysis

Three mechanisms of postoperative paralysis have been proposed: (1) parenchymal damage to the spinal cord caused by a rapid expansion in its volume accompanied by a sudden increase in blood flow; (2) an intradural tethering effect caused by the stretching of the intradural root filament by the dorsally shifted spinal cord (Fig. 4A); and (3) an extradural tethering

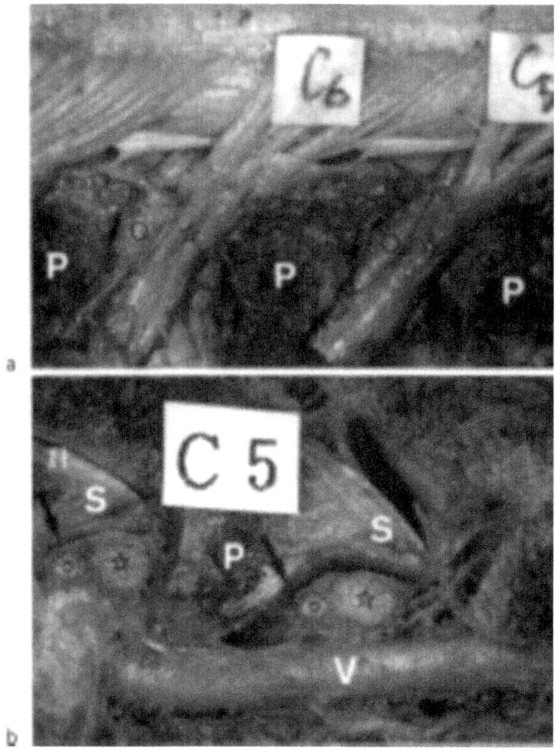

Fig. 2. Anatomy of a root inside an intervertebral foramen. Inside view of the intervertebral foramen of the cervical spine. **a** Posterior aspect after the removal of facets (*C5*, *C6*, C5 root and C6 root). **b** Sagittal aspect at the vertebral artery level (*C5*, lateral mass of the C5 vertebra). *P*, pedicle; *S*, superior articular process; *V*, vertebral artery; *circles*, anterior roots; *stars*, posterior root. For details see text (From [1], with permission)

effect caused by the traction on the extradural root by the expanded dura (Fig. 4b).

The expansion of the spinal cord which occurs after its release from compression usually produces beneficial effects on the parenchyma of the spinal cord, as manifested by neurological recovery. However, a sudden increase in blood flow might have some adverse effects on the devitalized motor cells. This might resemble the reperfusion syndrome after brain infarction, and this process might appear as a minor neurological dysfunction in the generally improved neurological functions. From this assumption, the theory of parenchyma injury has been proposed to explain the occurrence of motor dificits after decompression. The factors inducing paralysis might be the presence of free radicals, as observed after brain infarction, an excessive inflow of blood to already pathological motor cells, or venous congestion around the motor cells (see the chapter by K. Chiba in this volume). Although motor-dominant paralysis might be explained by this theory, which has some credibility, there is no definite evidence and it is still highly controversial. There are two main points of controversy (1) Why are only certain areas of the spinal cord affected while neighboring areas of identi-

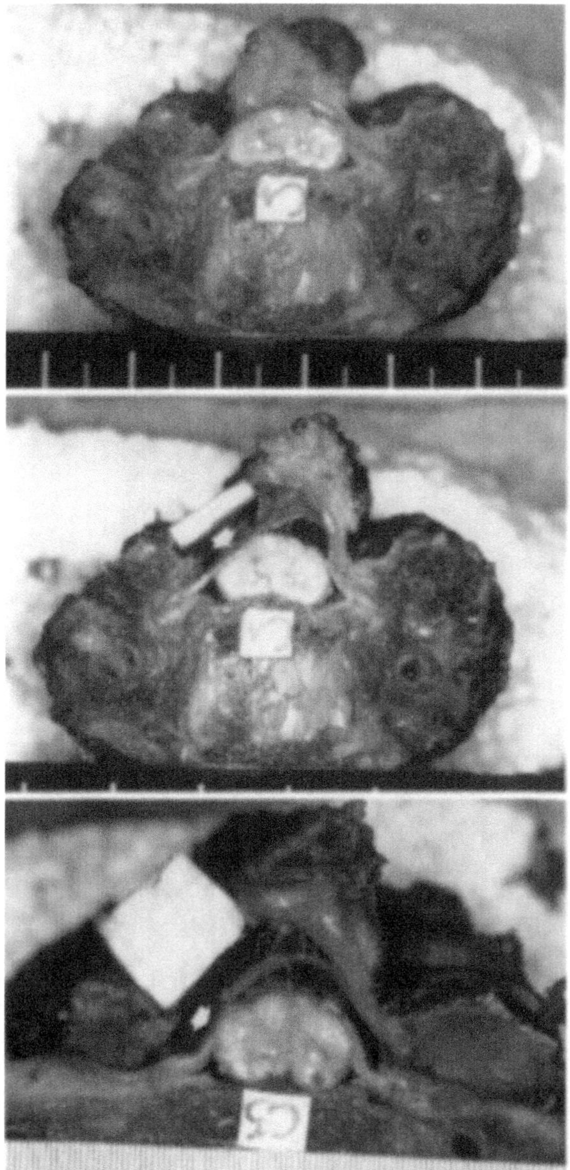

a

Fig. 3. Changes in dural tension after **a** posterior decompression, and **b** anterior decompression. **a**: *top*, before laminar decompression (laminar rotation); *center*, laminar rotation to increase dural tension through adhesion between the dura and the lamina (expanding the dura after decompression may also increase the dural tension); *bottom*, disappearance of the stretching force on the extradural portion of the root by longitudinal duratomy (*arrow*). **b**: *top*, before anterior decompression; *bottom*, after anterior decompression, the expanded anterior dura can stretch the anterior root (*arrow*). (Adapted from [1], with permission)

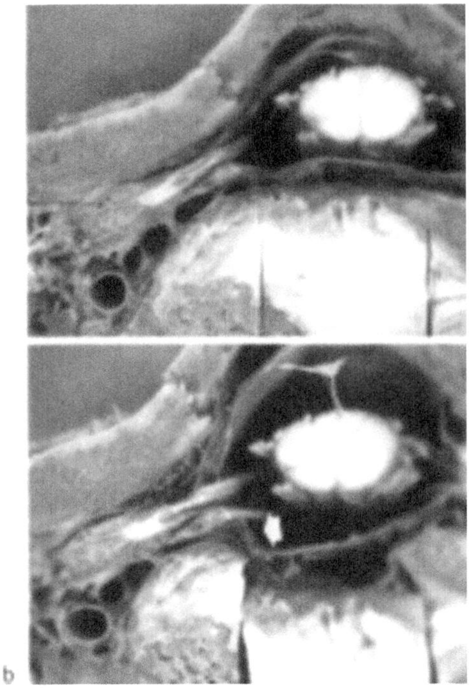

Fig. 3. *Continued*

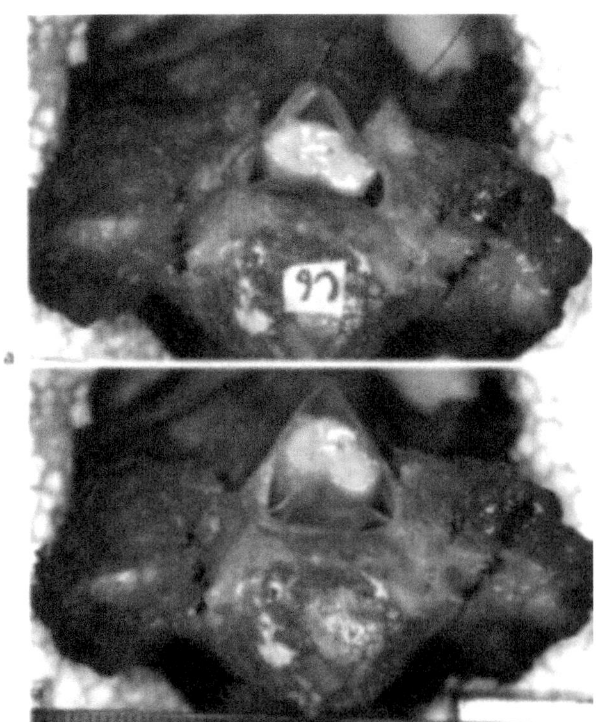

Fig. 4. Dural expansion after posterior decompression and changes in tension on the intra- and extradural portions of a root. In an expanded dural sac, the spinal cord moves back and forth with the pulsating movements of the cerebro spinal fluid. Therefore, the tension on the intradural roots changes between tense and relaxed conditions alternately. Conversely, the tension on the extradural roots is permanently increased (From [5])

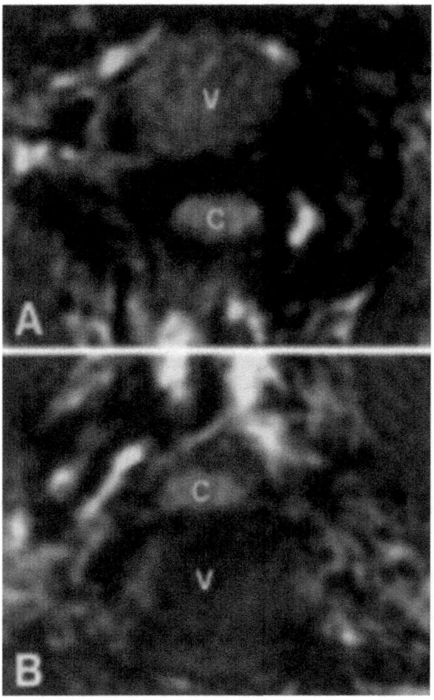

Fig. 5. The back and forth movements of the spinal cord due to gravity. Postoperative magnetic resonance images (MRIs) at the C5 level of a male patient, 50 years old, with severe unilateral postoperative C5 palsy. **A** The increase in the distance between the spinal cord (*C*) and the vertebral body (*V*) (*C–V* distance) in the supine position. **B** The decrease in the *C–V* distance in the prone position

cal pathology show an improvement? What is the explanation for the unilateral occurrence of paralysis, and the fact that long tracts of the spinal cord which might contain devitalized fibers are not involved? (2) Why does the frequency of occurrence differ according to the method of laminoplasty used in spite of almost identical degrees of spinal cord decompression?

The intradural tethering effect by the dorsally shifted spinal cord in the expanded dural sac, which has been assumed to be a major mechanism, may be less likely to cause paralysis because the intradural root filaments repeatedly elongate and relax following the back and forth movements of the spinal cord. These movements are generated by CSF pulsation or changes in gravity, and therefore the persistent stretched status that might induce nerve damage does not exist (Fig. 5). Anatomically, intradural root filaments are sufficiently long to clear the extension damage even when it reaches the full extent of the maximally expanded dural sac [5].

On the other hand, the extradural tethering effect is very likely to cause paralysis. The extradural portion of the roots is persistently stretched by the expanded dura (see Fig. 3a center). If this force is strong enough to cause root injury, postoperative paralysis of the arm might result. An anterior root is located in the narrowest portion of the intervertebral foramen, and a posterior root is in the relatively wider portion (see Fig. 2). If perineural fibrosis occurs around the anterior root, the ability of the roots to clear the stretching force may be less in the anterior root. Motor-dominant paralysis and the initial transient sensory irritation may be explained by these anatomic characteristics.

The degree of dural expansion by posterior decompression is greatest at the C4 and C5 level owing to the presence of cervical lordosis. This may explain the frequent occurrence of paralysis at the C5 root. The dural expanding force on the extradural roots disappears after longitudinal durotomy (see Fig. 3a, bottom). A controlled study of the effects of a longitudinal durotomy on the occurrence of postoperative paralysis resulted in a significant reduction in such paralysis ($P < 0.05$) [1]. In a case of severe postoperative C5 paralysis, the patient recovered after a longitudinal durotomy. The magnetic resonance imaging (MRI) findings in this case aroused controversy about the pathological significance of postoperative enlargement of the T2 high lesion in the spinal cord (Fig. 6).

The existence of paralysis of radicular origin has been supported by extensive clinical evidences, but the possibility that paralysis is caused by spinal cord parenchymal damage cannot be ruled out and needs further study.

Methods of Prevention and Treatment

During a laminoplasty, a position that will reduce root tension (a crouching position) is recommended [6] to place the bony gutter on the medial side of the zygoapophyseal joint and to maintain the slope of the opened lamina within 60° [2, 7]. In cases of postoperative paralysis, if it is caused by parenchymal damage to the spinal cord, then nothing can be done except to a wait the outcome. However, at present there is no way of knowing whether the paralysis is caused by parenchymal damage. Although MRI findings may be the key to assessing parenchymal changes in the spinal cord, no reliable hard ware for checking the degree of parenchymal damage is available at present. Therefore, the presence of an extradural tethering effect, which might be relieved by appropriate methods, should be checked. The first step is to check for the presence of tenderness by a fingertip placed on the root foramen corresponding to the paralysis. If this indicates severe tenderness on the root, or induces radicular pain, 5–10 ml of diluted anesthetic (we use 0.5% xylocaine), with or without a steroid, should be injected in to the subcutaneous space over the foramen and rubbed in with a fingertip. If this maneuver reduces the pain or increases the muscle power, the presence of an extradural tethering effect should be considered. The arm should then be held in a position which reduces root tension (hand-on-chest position) by a sling, and the injection should be repeated once as twice a week for about 1 month.

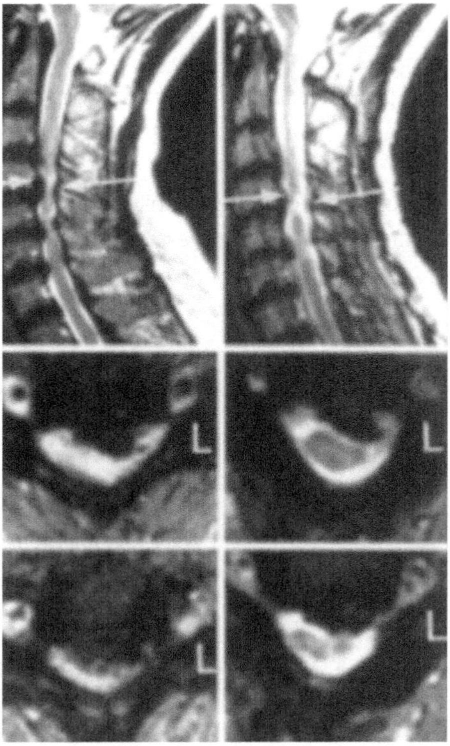

Fig. 6. MRI findings in a female patient, 57 years old, who recovered from C5 palsy after longitudinal durotomy. The patient had cervical ossification of the posterior longitudinal ligament compressing the spinal cord at the C4–C5 vertebral levels. Immediately after posterior decompression by open-door laminoplasty (left-side opening), the left C5–C8 root-innervated muscles showed complete motor loss. Several hours later, a spontaneous recovery of muscle power occurred in the C7 and C8 muscles. For persistent C5 muscle weakness (manual muscle testing (MMT) score 0), a longitudinal durotomy was performed on the day after the operation. Immediately after durotomy, the C5 muscle recovered to MMT 3. After 1 year, the patient's MMT scores were: 5 for the C5 muscle; 4 for the C6 muscle; 5 for the C7 and C8 muscles. Although postoperative MRI showed an increase and enlargement of the T2 high shadow at the C4 vertebral level, this phenomenon seemed to bear no relation to the occurrence of postoperative paralysis in this patient. *Left*, preoperative MRIs (2 months before the operation): *top*, sagittal view; *center*, axial view corresponding to the proximal arrow in the top picture; *bottom*, axial view corresponding to the inferior arrow in the top picture. *Right*, postoperative MRIs (3 months after the operation): *top*, sagittal view; *center*, axial view corresponding to the proximal arrow in the top picture; *bottom*, axial view corresponding to the inferior arrow in the top picture

Prognosis

If the patient's motor power on MMT is above 2, a spontaneous recovery to a useful level with in 3–12 months is the most common outcome. If severe paralysis persists, i.e., an MMT score of 0 or 1, a longitudinal durotomy might be considered, or appropriate reconstructive surgery may be indicated if a significant dysfunction of the arm persists.

References

1. Tsuzuki N, Abe R, Saiki K, et al. (1996) Extradural tethering effect as one mechanism of radiculopathy complicating posterior decompression of the cervical spinal cord. Spine 21:203–211
2. Uematsu Y, Tokuhashi Y, Matsuzaki H (1998) Radiculopathy after laminoplasty of the cervical spine. Spine 23:2057–2062
3. Shimizu K, Shimada H, Edakuni H (1996) Post-laminoplasty palsy of upper extremities, with special reference to the spinal cord factors. Bessatsu-Seikeigeka 29:188–194
4. Frykholm R (1951) Lower cervical roots and their investments. Acta Chir Scand 101: 457–471
5. Tsuzuki N, Li Z, Abe R, et al. (1993) Paralysis of the arm after posterior decompression of the cervical spinal cord. I. Anatomical investigation of the mechanism of paralysis. Eur Spine J 2:191–196
6. Epstein JA (1996) Letter to the Editor. Spine 21:1839–1841
7. Tsuzuki N, Abe R, Saiki K, et al. (1993) Paralysis of the arm after posterior decompression of the cervical spinal cord. II. Analysis of clinical findings. Eur Spine J 2: 197–202

Segmental Motor Paralysis After Laminoplasty

Kazuhiro Chiba, Hirofumi Maruiwa, Morio Matsumoto, and Yoshiaki Toyama

Since the introduction of the simultaneous decompression technique using a high-speed drill, the incidence of neurological complications after posterior decompression has dramatically decreased. However, although not frequent, complications characteristic of laminoplasty, such as axial pain and segmental motor paralysis that mainly involve the C5 segment, have evolved [1, 2].

The incidence of segmental paralysis has been reported to lie between 4% and 13% of surgical cases after a variety of laminoplasties [3–11]. The paralysis usually occurs several days after surgery, and is often preceded by a sharp tingling pain in the neck and shoulder. Deltoid and biceps brachii muscles innervated by the C5 segment are most frequently affected, but sensory disturbance of the segment involved is absent in most cases. The prognosis of the paralysis is usually good, with spontaneous regression within 1–2 years [11].

The occurrence of this paralysis has long been attributed to nerve root lesions due to premature techniques including the mishandling of surgical instruments such as high-speed drills and Kerrison rongeurs, and excessive drilling of the hinge gutter resulting in the detachment of the laminar door (Fig. 1) [1, 5, 6].

However, the incidence of paralysis, did not drop substantially although a number of improvements had been made in the surgical techniques. It even occurred frequently in the hinge side without the presence of hinge detachment, as shown on postoperative computed tomography (CT) scans.

The tethering effect on the nerve root induced by an excessive posterior shift of the spinal cord, or an impingement on the stretched nerve root at the resected end of the laminae are other possible explanations that are sup-

Department of Orthopaedic Surgery, School of Medicine, Keio University, 35 Shinanomachi, Shinjuku-ku, Tokyo 160-8582, Japan

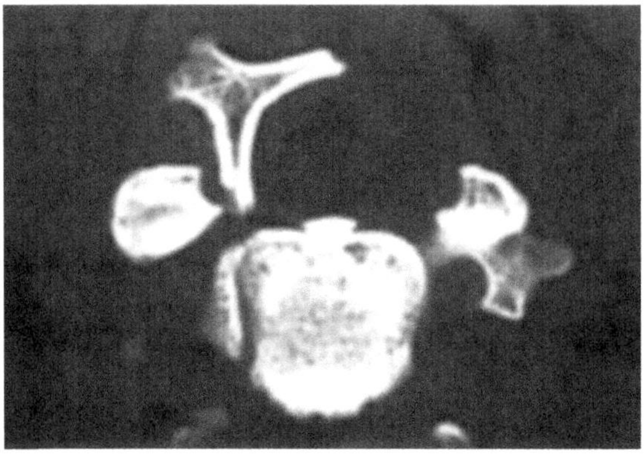

Fig. 1. Fracture and detachment of the laminar hinge due to excessive drilling of the hinge gutter

ported by a number of investigators [1, 2, 5, 9, 10, 12, 13]. Several measures such as foraminotomy, facetectomy, and durotomy have been suggested as ways to relieve the tension of the nerve roots, thereby reducing its incidence [9]. Uematsu et al. [10] also suggested that the prevention of extensive opening of the laminar door may lead to a reduction in the incidence of paralysis. However, the exact etiology of this paralysis still remains unclear, and definite preventive measures have not been established to date.

Our recent study on 208 patients who underwent ELAP between 1993 and 1998 revealed that segmental paralysis developed in 16 patients, giving an overall incidence of 7.7% (16/208) [3]. A detailed analysis of 15 patients who were observed for more than 2 years postoperatively revealed that the paralysis was detected mainly, at the C5 segment, but was not confined to that segment, and eight patients had multisegment involvement. The paralysis occurred predominantly in the hinge side (10 patients), and there were two patients with bilateral involvement. The paralysis developed after a short delay (mean 4.6 days). Ten out of 15 patients complained of severe numbness and dysesthesia in their upper extremities, and their upper extremity sensory disturbance was more pronounced than their long tract motor signs, including gait disturbance and clumsiness of finger motions. The average recovery rate of the upper extremity sensory disturbance was significantly lower in patients with paralysis than those without paralysis, although overall neurological recovery was not significantly different between the two patient populations. Postoperative cervical alignment did not affect the incidence of paralysis. Preoperative magnetic resonance (MR) images of the paralyzed patients showed severe spinal cord compression that was not proportional to the relatively mild long tract signs in all patients. It is noteworthy that postoperative MR images revealed the presence of T2 high-signal-intensity zones in the spinal cord, mostly in the central gray matter, in all 15 patients (Fig. 2). The locations of the high-intensity signals

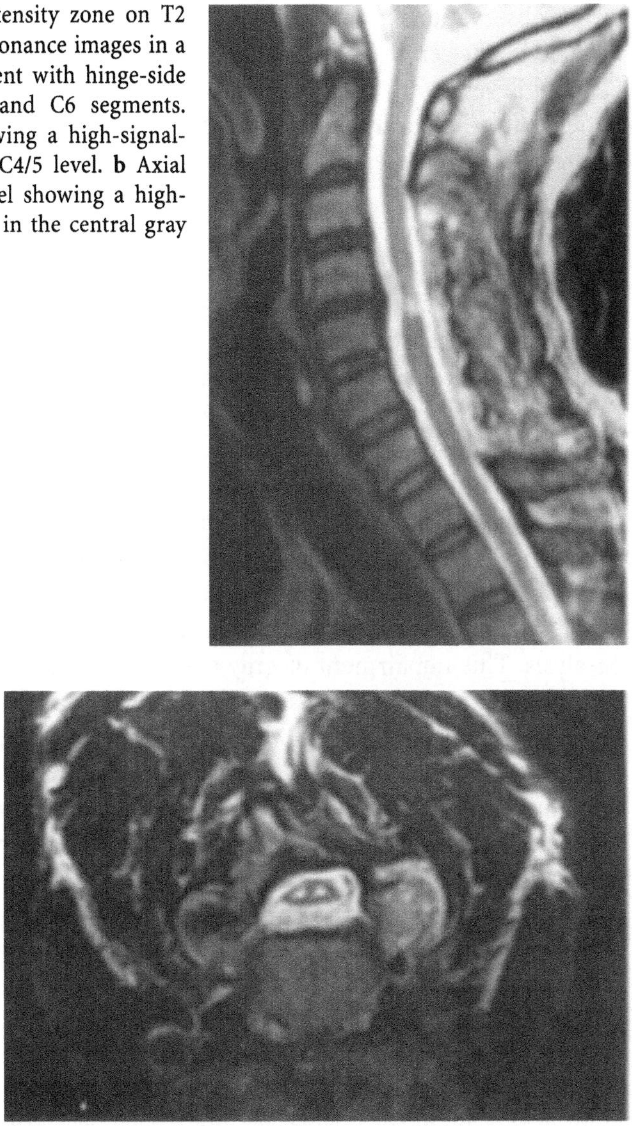

Fig. 2. High-signal-intensity zone on T2 weighted magnetic resonance images in a 46-year-old male patient with hinge-side paralysis in the C5 and C6 segments. **a** Saggital image showing a high-signal-intensity zone at the C4/5 level. **b** Axial image at the C4/5 level showing a high-intensity zone located in the central gray matter

corresponded well to the levels of the paralyzed segments, as proposed by Tsuzuki [14], in 12 of the 15 patients. No dislodging of the hinge or reclosure of the laminae were found in these patients. The paralysis resolved completely in 11 patients, while a mild motor weakness of grade 4 in manual muscle testing (MMT) remained in four patients. Patients with a sequela tended to have larger high-signal-intensity zones, which had not regressed on follow-up MR images.

The observations in our study, e.g., (1) the incidence of paralysis was not affected by the cervical alignment or the causes of spinal cord compression, (2) multilevel paralysis was found in more than half of the paralyzed patients, (3) the paralysis occurred after a short delay, and (4) no sensory disturbance was present in the concomitant segment in the majority of the cases, suggest that the mechanical injuries to the nerve root, including traumatic surgical techniques and the tethering effect alone, cannot fully explain the occurrence of this paralysis. If the root injury is the cause, sensory disturbance should be present in the concomitant segments, and if the tethering effect is the cause, the incidence of paralysis should be higher in patients with cervical lordosis and in patients with massive OPLL, in whom the spinal cord is expected to shift further posteriorly.

The other interesting findings of our study, such as the presence of severe numbness and dysesthesia in the upper extremities, resembling that observed in patients with central spinal cord injury, the poor recovery of such upper extremity sensory disturbance after surgery, and the presence of T2 high-signal zones in the central gray matter suggest that an impairment of the gray matter may play a role in the development of segmental motor paralysis. This impairment of gray matter, which could manifest itself as a T2 high-intensity zone on postoperative MR images, may represent changes in the microcirculation within the spinal cord. An underlying long-standing impairment in the blood flow in the spinal cord due to chronic severe compression followed by acute reperfusion and hyperemia after decompression may have led to edema, which could further damage the gray matter and eventually cause paralysis.

Damage to the nerve tissues may be caused by a rapid rise in pO_2 in the early stage of reperfusion in the hypoxic tissues, inducing a risk of oxidative cell injury from the formation of free radicals and other toxic products of oxidative reactions [15]. Rapid calcium entry into the cells during reperfusion could be another explanation of this injury [16].

Shimizu et al., in 1996 [7], were the first to suggest the possible involvement of the spinal cord. However, there have been few studies to test their hypothesis of spinal cord involvement. The results of our study further support the possible involvement of spinal cord pathology as a cause of this paralysis.

The etiology of segmental motor paralysis after ELAP may be multifactorial, and in addition to nerve root pathology, the impairment of the spinal cord autoregulation may be an important factor in the development of the segmental paralysis.

The prophylactic use of antioxidative drugs such as superoxide dismutase, and calcium entry blockers such as verapamil, and the application of hypotensive anesthesia at the time of laminar opening may be an effective way to prevent some cases of this paralysis [16–18]. The feasibility and efficacy of such measures need to be extensively evaluated in future studies.

References

1. Hirabayashi K, Satomi K (1988) Operative procedure and results of expansive open-door laminoplasty. Spine 13:870–876
2. Satomi K, Nishi Y, Kohno T, et al. (1994) Long-term follow-up studies of open-door expansive laminoplasty for cervical stenotic myelopathy. Spine 19:507–510
3. Chiba K, Watanabe M, Maruiwa H, et al. (2000) Segmental motor paralysis after expansive open-door laminoplasty for cervical myelopathy. (in Japanese) Rinsho Seikeigeka 35:607–612
4. Ebara S, Yonenobu K, Fujiwara K, et al. (1987) Neurological complications after surgical treatment for cervical radiculopathy and myelopathy. (in Japanese) Rinsho Seikeigeka 22:802–810
5. Iwamoto Y, Fujimura Y, Nishi Y, et al. (1996) Neurological complications in early stage after expansive open-door laminoplasty. (in Japanese) Bessatsu Seikeigeka 29:200–204
6. Osawa Y, Takeuchi N, Makino N, et al. (1996) Surgical technique for preventing neurological complications in open-door laminoplasty. (in Japanese) Bessatsu Seikeigeka 29:205–209
7. Shimizu T, Shimada H, Edakuni H (1996) Post-laminoplasty palsy of upper extremities, with special reference to the spinal cord factors. (in Japanese) Bessatsu Seikeigeka 29:188–193
8. Tokuhashi Y, Matsuzaki H, Wakabayashi K (1996) Postoperative cervical radiculopathy after laminoplasty. (in Japanese) Bessatsu Seikeigeka 29:195–199
9. Tsuzuki N, Abe R, Saiki K, et al. (1996) Extradural tethering effect as one mechanism of radiculopathy complicating posterior decompression of the cervical spinal cord. Spine 21:203–211
10. Uematsu Y, Tokuhashi Y, Matsuzaki H (1998) Radiculopathy after laminoplasty of the cervical spine. Spine 23:2057–2062
11. Yonenobu K, Yamamoto T, Ono K (1998) Laminoplasty for myelopathy indications, results, outcome, and complications. In: CSRS Editorial Committee (eds) The cervical spine. 3rd edn. Lippincott-Raven, Philadelphia, pp 849–864
12. Hirabayashi K, Toyama Y, Chiba K (1999) Expansive laminoplasty for myelopathy in ossification of the longitudinal ligament. Clin Orthop 359:35–48
13. Yonenobu K, Hosono N, Iwasaki M, et al. (1991) Neurologic complications of surgery for cervical compression myelopathy. Spine 16:1277–1282
14. Tsuzuki N (1993) Topographical relation of cervical spinal cord segments to cervical vertebrae (in Japanese). Spine Spinal Cord 6:401–406
15. Kim-Lee MH, Stokes BT, Yates AJ (1992) Reperfusion paradox: a novel mode of glial cell injury. Glia 5:56–64
16. Chavko M, Kalincakova K, Kluchova D, et al. (1991) Blood flow and electrolytes in spinal cord ischemia. Exp Neurol 112:299–303
17. Agee JM, Flanagan T, Blackbourne LH, et al. (1991) Reducing postischemic paraplegia using conjugated superoxide dismutase. Ann Thorac Surg 51:911–914
18. Wisselink W, Money SR, Crockett DE, et al. (1994) Ischemia-reperfusion injury of the spinal cord: protective effect of the hydroxyl radical scavenger dimethylthiourea. J Vasc Surg 20:444–491

Cervical Pain After Cervical Laminoplasty: Causes and Treatments

Kazuo Saita and Yuichi Hoshino

Introduction

A number of studies have reported on the satisfactory results of cervical laminoplasty for cervical spondylotic myelopathy (CSM) and ossification of the posterior longitudinal ligament (OPLL) [1–4]. Because of its good results and low morbidity compared with anterior decompression surgery [5], laminoplasty has become the standard procedure for multisegmental cord compression in the cervical region. There is excellent neurological recovery after cervical laminoplasty, but many patients complain about postoperative neck pain or tension as well as shoulder stiffness. In the first report on axial pain, Hosono et al. [6] noted that 60% of patients suffered from neck and shoulder symptoms following unilateral open-type laminoplasty. In recent publications, there are few studies of patients' postoperative complaints, although these report many examples of patients' satisfaction with the treatment. Therefore, an open discussion about postoperational pain is needed. Complaints about postoperative neck troubles involve not only occasional discomfort, but also cases of pain or stiffness requiring regular massage, local injection therapy, or medication. Flexion of the cervical vertebrae aggravates the symptoms in many patients, hindering their ability to work for a long time at a desk, or even making it impossible to return to work. As most of the complaints involve patients' own perception, their verification by an objective examination of symptoms is difficult. Generally speaking, patients complain about stiffness, tension, or pain in the region from the nucha to the trapezius muscle, and sometimes also involving the interscapulum. Pain may impair the middle or lateral portion, as well as the whole region. In addition, cervical troubles can be unilateral or bilateral. There are

Department of Orthopaedic Surgery, Jichi Medical School, 3311-1 Yakushiji, Minamikawachi-machi, Kawachi-gun, Tochigi 329-0498, Japan also cases of pain being aggravated at a change of season or during a rainy period. Except for unilateral cases, complaints about postoperative pain are similar to symptoms of cervical distortion. In some patients, the symptoms are aggravated after long-lasting cervical flexion. In clinics, only a few cases of movement- or pressure-related pain have been seen. Sometimes, pain can occur in paravertebral muscles, or be localized on the internal scapular line. Cervical mobility is impaired after the operation in many cases, but there are no extreme differences between patients complaining about nuchal discomfort. Generally speaking, serious complaints about self-awareness of cervical discomfort with a lack of objective clinical symptoms are specific to each patient. Some of the possible factors causing postoperative cervical pain which have been reported to date include cervical flexion, mobility, operation range and time, expansion degree, and muscular or neural injury. The most important research on these possibilities are reviewed here.

Reviews

Saita et al. [7] observed 83 patients after French-window open-type cervical laminoplasty. In this method, which was developed by Kurokawa, splitting of the spinous process is performed along the sagittal axis. This is followed by an asymmetrical approach as one side of the trapezius muscle is dissected from the midline septum just lateral to the nuchal ligament. The patients were divided into groups according to their degree of pain: (1) pain (–), i.e., those who had no symptoms; (2) treatment (–), i.e., those who complained of cervical pain but did not require treatment; (3) treatment (+), i.e., those who complained of cervical pain and required treatment. Three months after their operation, 27 patients were classified as pain (–), 34 as treatment (–), and 22 as treatment (+). Operation time was one of the factors examined, and was found to be statistically significantly correlated with postoperative cervical pain. For other categories such as gender, disease, age, method of muscle reconstruction, and intraoperative blood loss there was no such correlation. As muscular injury is known to correlate with the time that pressure lasts, it could be suggested that this correlation with operation time could be the result of intraoperative injury of the dorsal muscles. In addition, the side of the cervical pain was consistent with the side of the surgical approach in 29 cases, inconsistent in 7 cases, and bilateral in 20 cases. During this operation, soft tissues are dissected asymmetrically, whereas the laminae are expanded symmetrically. It is unlikely that symmetrical bone cutting could result in complaints of asymmetrical cervical pain. The relationship between the localization of pain and the side of the surgical approach suggests that intraoperative injury of soft tissues could be the most important cause of postoperative cervical pain. Both the laterality and the time coincidence suggest that damage to the posterior neck muscles from compression by a retractor causes cervical pain.

Fujimura and Nishi [8] observed postoperative atrophy in nuchal muscles using C4/5 computed tomography (CT) scans. Measured values showed that atrophy occurred in 20% of the patients. In addition, atrophy of deep nuchal muscles which was correlated with lordosis has also been reported.

Oohori et al. [9] analyzed C5/6 magnetic resonance imaging (MRI) postoperative scans and compared them with the scans taken before the operation. They found that atrophy of posterior cervical muscles occurs in 20% of complaining patients, compared with 10% atrophy occurrence in noncomplaining patients. This report concluded that there is a correlation between atrophy of the nuchal muscles and axial pain.

Yokoyama et al. [10] reported that intraoperative muscular injury and impairment of circulation might cause complaints of cervical pain. They observed the postoperative progress of 30 patients for a period of 1 year. The criteria for cervical complaints were as follows: no pain or mild pain accompanying movement, no pressure-related pain, aggravation by warmth and improvement by cold, and no pain if lying on one's back. The patients were divided into two groups according to the severity of their complaints, and, independently of this grouping, into other groups according to the impairment of their activities of daily living (ADL) or their inability to work because of nuchal troubles. MRI (T1 axial view) scans taken at C5 or C5/6 in 21 patients were used to calculate the nuchal muscular area and the severity of its postoperative decrease. In 11 of the patients complaining of postoperative cervical discomfort, 37% had severe disease. There was a significant correlation with operation time, since in mildly impaired patients it was 2 h 43 ± 59 min, whereas in severely impaired patients it was 3 h 40 ± 36 min. No correlation was found with other factors such as CSM or OPLL, preoperative Japanese Orthopaedic Association (JOA) score, preoperative cervicovertebral alignment, preoperative cervical mobility, duration of postoperative collar insertion, postoperative cervicovertebral alignment, or postoperative cervical mobility. The decrease in the cross-sectional areas of muscles was significantly different between mildly impaired patients with 10.5 ± 6.0% ($n = 12$) and severely impaired patients with 21.6 ± 6.3% ($n = 9$). From the correlation between operation time and degree of muscular atrophy, the authors concluded that protracted use of a retractor could cause intraoperative muscular injury and circulatory impairment, with consequent cervical complaints.

In 1999 Kawaguchi et al. [11] suggested that not only muscular injury but also a decrease in cervical mobility could be a possible cause of postoperative pain. They analyzed 82 patients after unilateral open-type en bloc cervical laminoplasty. As they expected the formation of synostosis in the enlarged part, they inserted an orthosis for 3 postoperative months. After the operation, the patients filled in a questionnaire concerning their axial symptoms. They were divided into groups according to their neck pain and/or stiffness, and ADL. Axial complaints were made by 80% patients, but there was no difference in JOA score between the complaining and uncomplaining group. A significant correlation was found between severe pain and long operational time. A strong, but not significant, correlation was found between intraoperative bleeding and postoperative creatine phosphokinase (CPK) activity. Mobility was decreased in the severely impaired group, and in particular the chin–chest distance measured in cervical flexion and extension was significantly smaller. In addition, X-rays revealed fused laminae, with consequent decreased cervical mobility, significantly more frequently in severely impaired patients. It was concluded that decreased mobility due to the impairment of paravertebral muscles, as well as spontaneous fusion of laminae, are causes of postoperative cervical complaints.

Mochida et al. [12] suggested that, in addition to muscular injury, cervicovertebral alignment might also play an important role. They pulled the spinous process of C7 toward the caudal site to be approximately against the lateral aspect of the spinous process of T1. The ends of the spinous process from C4 to C7 were sutured to the nuchal ligament on the hinged side to improve the reconstruction of soft tissues. As a result, tension in the nuchal ligament became strong and maintained cervical lordosis. The application of an hydroxy apatite HA spacer in open-type cervical laminoplasty reduced postoperative complaints to 7 out of 70 patients. There was no significant difference between pre- and postoperative range of motion (ROM), and CT scans did not show any important muscular fatty degeneration or atrophy. As the previous occurrence of postoperative cervical pain was 24%, the authors concluded that this method could be useful to reduce cervical pain. Moreover, they calculated that less injury to the posterior muscles at the hinge side, well-maintained segmental stability, and sagittal vertebral alignment are the mechanisms underlying the reduction of postoperative cervical pain.

Intraoperative damage to innervation is also thought to be an important cause of postoperative pain. In an anatomical study, Tsuzuki [13] showed that expansion of the vertebral arch damages posterior branches of the cervical nerve, with consequent atrophy of the cervical semispinalis as well as the multifidus muscle. In addition, he showed that an injury to intervertebral joints might be another cause of cervical pain. Dweyer et al. [14] studied the relationship between the innervation or stimulation of intervertebral joints and pain localization which is similar to cervical pain after cervical laminoplasty.

Postoperative care is another factor which is thought to be important. Kiya et al. [15] observed the progress after 1 year of 24 patients who had used postoperative orthotic fixation for 2 months after the operation, and 19 patients who had not had any fixation. More than half of the patients with fixation had pain of at least middle-grade intensity, whereas only mild pain was experienced by the patients without fixation, and this had stopped within 3 months. Moreover, cervical mobility was well maintained in patients without fixation. Hayashi et al. [16] compared 130 patients with orthotic fixation lasting 12-weeks with 60 patients with fixation in place for 6 weeks; 21.7% of the patients with 12-weeks fixation had cervical pain requiring treatment for more than 6 months. In contrast, 8.3% of patients without fixation had pain requiring some therapy. In addition, in the group with the longer-lasting fixation, the decrease in mobility was more serious. All of the reports mentioned above concluded that postoperative orthotic fixation is harmful and causes cervical pain.

Discussion

Cervical pain after vertebral laminoplasty clearly correlates with the patient's satisfaction with the treatment, but its causes, as well as countermeasures needed, are still being evaluated. As cervical pain has many causes, there is a strong probability that pain after cervical laminoplasty can also have multiple causes. Previous reports clearly show that there is no common cause, and that each of the factors considered could play an independent role. What is common to all these reports is that postoperative cervical pain correlates well with operational time and a decrease in cervical mobility. As the various surgical techniques reported to date differ in detail, although all of them share operational time-dependency, it can be hypothesized that the operation time itself, or some procedure resulting in its prolongation, causes postoperative cervical pain. On the other hand, if there are serious pathological changes in intervertebral joints, their extension will require a longer time and also a wider approach. What is the real cause and what is only a consequent result should be studied intensively. The same can be said about cervical mobility, as there is the clear possibility that pain causes a decrease in mobility. The short-term application of fixation is known to improve postoperative cervical pain, and therefore patients often demand it. Moreover, there is no evidence that 1–2 weeks fixation is harmful to mobility, although many cases have been analyzed. Reported results only describe clinical experience, and therefore cannot be generalized. Cervical laminoplasty is a very frequent operation, and therefore countermeasures to prevent postoperative cervical pain will dramatically improve patient satisfaction with this operation.

References

1. Hirabayashi K, Satomi K (1988) Operative procedure and results of expansive open-door laminoplasty. Spine 13:870–876
2. Kawai S, Sunaga K, Doi K, et al. (1988) Cervical laminoplasty (Hattori's method). Spine 13:1245–1250
3. Kimura I, Shingu H, Nasu Y (1995) Long-term follow-up of cervical spondylotic myelopathy treated by canal-expansive laminoplasty. J Bone Joint Surg Br 77:956–961
4. Satomi K, Nishi Y, Kohno T, et al. (1994) Long-term follow-up studies of open-door expansive laminoplasty for cervical stenotic myelopathy. Spine 19:507–510
5. Yonenobu K, Hosono N, Iwasaki M, et al. (1992) Laminoplasty versus subtotal corpectomy. Spine 17:1281–1284
6. Hosono N, Yonenobu K, Ono K (1996) Neck pain and shoulder pain after laminoplasty. Spine 21: 1969–1973
7. Saita K, Hoshino Y, Kikkawa I, et al. (1999) Complaint of nuchal pain following cervical laminoplasty. J Musculoskeletal Res 3:253–258
8. Fujimura Y, Nishi Y (1996) Atrophy of the nuchal muscle and change in cervical curvature after expansive open-door laminoplasty. Arch Orthop Trauma Surg 115: 203–205
9. Oohori Y, Asaduma T, Iso K, et al. (1998) Post-operative neck pain after expansive laminoplasty (abstract, in Japanese). J Jpn Spine Res Soc 9:260
10. Yokoyama T, Harata S, Ueyama K, et al. (2001) Risk factor for chronic pain after cervical laminoplasty. In: Investigation committee report on the ossification of the spinal ligament (in Japanese). Japanese Ministry of Public Health and Welfare in 2000, Tokyo, pp 153–155
11. Kawaguchi Y, Matsui H, Ishihara H, et al. (1999) Axial symptoms after en bloc cervical laminoplasty. J Spinal Disord 12:392–395
12. Mochida J, Nomura T, Chiba M, et al. (1999) Modified expansive open-door laminoplasty in cervical myelopathy. J Spinal Disord 12:386–391
13. Tsuzuki N (2000) Problems related to the posterior decompression of the cervical spinal cord for cervical myelopathy, mainly from the results of cervical laminoplasty (in Japanese). J Jpn Orthop Assoc 74:1–10
14. Dweyer A, Aprill C, Bogduk N (1990) Cervical zygapophysial joint pain patterns. 1. A study in normal volunteers. Spine 15:453–457
15. Kiya T, Nohara Y, Tomura T, et al. (1998) The effectiveness of early isometric muscle exercise without collar fixation after cervical laminoplasty (abstract, in Japanese). J Jpn Spine Res Soc 9:259
16. Hayashi M, Ito Y, Goto F, et al. (1998) Postoperative immobilization and neck pain after cervical expansive laminoplasty (abstract, in Japanese). J Jpn Spine Res Soc 9:261

Neck and Shoulder Pain: Postoperative Neck Pain with Special Reference to Postoperative Immobilization

YUTAKA NOHARA and TETSURO KIYA

Introduction

Laminoplasty has achieved good results in the treatment of cervical myelopathy. However, some patients whose spinal symptoms have been relieved by laminoplasty have suffered from new axial symptoms such as neck pain and stiffness of the neck and shoulder muscles after surgery.

Yonenobu et al. [1] have noted discomfort of the neck and a reduction in the range of motion (ROM) of the cervical spine as disadvantages of laminoplasty. Since 1984, we have performed extensive simultaneous multisegment laminectomy and posterolateral fusion, the so-called Kirita–Miyazaki method [2]. We have experienced occasional cases of kyphotic deformity and neck pain due to weakened posterior supporting tissue, and also a severe reduction in the ROM of the cervical spine after the surgery (Fig. 1). Consequently, since 1992 we have conducted spinous process splitting laminoplasty, the so-called Kurokawa method [3], which allows reconstruction of the posterior supporting tissue using ceramic laminal spacers, and reattachment of posterior muscles in order to prevent kyphotic deformity. Patients who underwent either type of laminoplasty wore a Philadelphia collar for 2 months after surgery, as usual. Later, however, long-term external fixation was considered to induce joint and muscular contracture and/or muscular atrophy, resulting in a deleterious effect on alignment and a reduction in the ROM in the cervical spine. Consequently, since 1996 we have started posture exercises, ROM exercises, and muscle-strengthening exercises immediately after surgery without external fixation (Fig. 2). However, some patients have complained of axial symptoms even after these changes to the surgical procedure and postoperative management were made (Fig. 3).

Department of Orthopaedic Surgery, Koshigaya Hospital, School of Medicine, Dokkyo University, 2-1-50 Minami-Koshigaya, Koshigaya, Saitama 343-8555, Japan

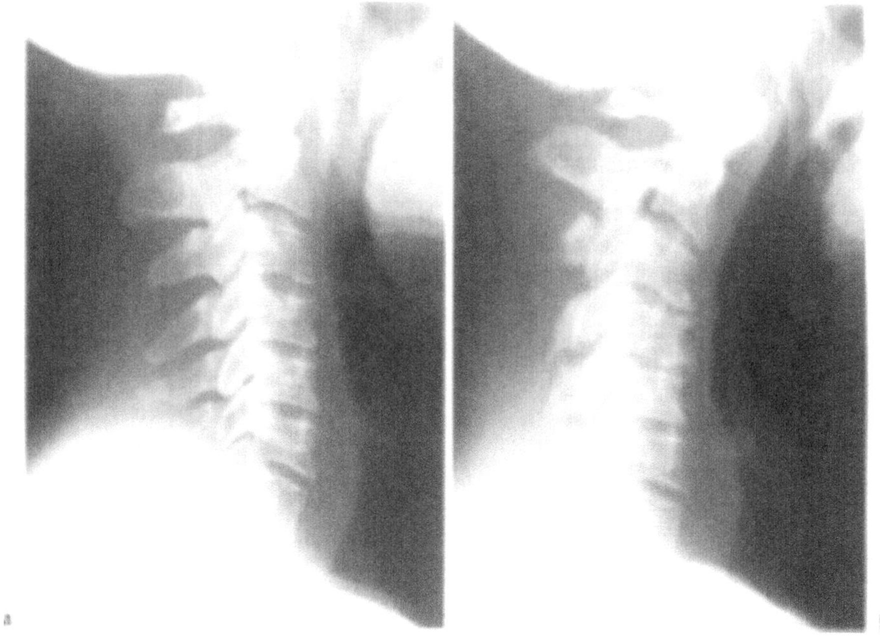

Fig. 1. A 52-year-old man was treated by laminoplasty (Kirita–Miyazaki method) for cervical spondylotic myelopathy. **a** Preoperative X-ray showing an almost normal alignment of the cervical spine. **b** Two years after the operation, an X-ray showed severe kyphotic deformity of the cervical spine. The patient complains of severe neck pain and needs analgesics every day

Are axial symptoms really caused by laminoplasty? We investigated the differences among three groups which had different methods of laminoplasty and/or postoperative management.

Materials and Methods

A total of 188 patients with cervical myelopathy underwent laminoplasty at Koshigaya Hospital, Dokkyo University, from 1984 to 1998. We evaluated 108 patients who could be followed for a minimum of 2 years (range 2–16 years), and excluded 80 cases with spinal injuries as well as anterior fusion. The average age at surgery was 57 years (range 20–75 years), 84 patients were male, and 24 were female. Their diagnoses were 50 cases of cervical spondylotic myelopathy, and 58 cases of ossification of the posterior longitudinal ligament. Forty-three cases were treated by the Kirita–Miyazaki method (group A), and 65 cases by the Kurokawa method. Eighteen of these 65 cases had a fixed collar after surgery (group B). The remaining 47 cases were

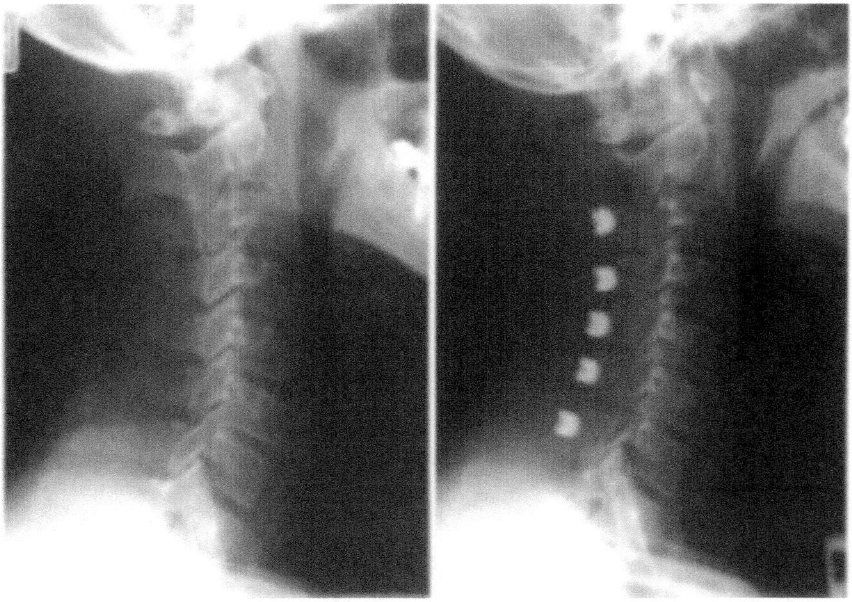

a b

Fig. 2. A 61-year-old man was treated by laminoplasty (Kurokawa method) for cervical spondylotic myelopathy. **a** Preoperative X-ray showing a narrow spinal canal of the cervical spine. **b** Two years after surgery, an X-ray showed no kyphotic deformity of the cervical spine. The patient's myelopathic symptoms had been relieved and he has no postoperative axial symptoms

treated by the Kurokawa method, and no external fixation was used after surgery (group C) (Table 1).

In this investigation, we focused on three risk factors for axial symptoms in relation to the changes in surgical procedure and postoperative treatment. These factors were preoperative neck pain, kyphotic deformity, and restricted ROM (<70%) of the cervical spine 1 year after laminoplasty. Since it was difficult to evaluate neck or shoulder pain objectively, patients who used analgesics were taken to be those with pain.

Results (Table 2)

Postoperative neck pain had resolved within a few months after laminoplasty in the majority of patients. We found that only 9% (4 cases) of cases in group A, 11% (2 cases) in group B, and 4% (2 cases) in group C had persistent neck pain for more than 2 years. Thirteen cases in group A, 6 cases in group B, and 10 cases in group C had preoperative neck pain. Three cases in group A had postoperative kyphotic deformity, but no postoperative kyphotic deformity was observed in groups B and C. Thirteen cases in group

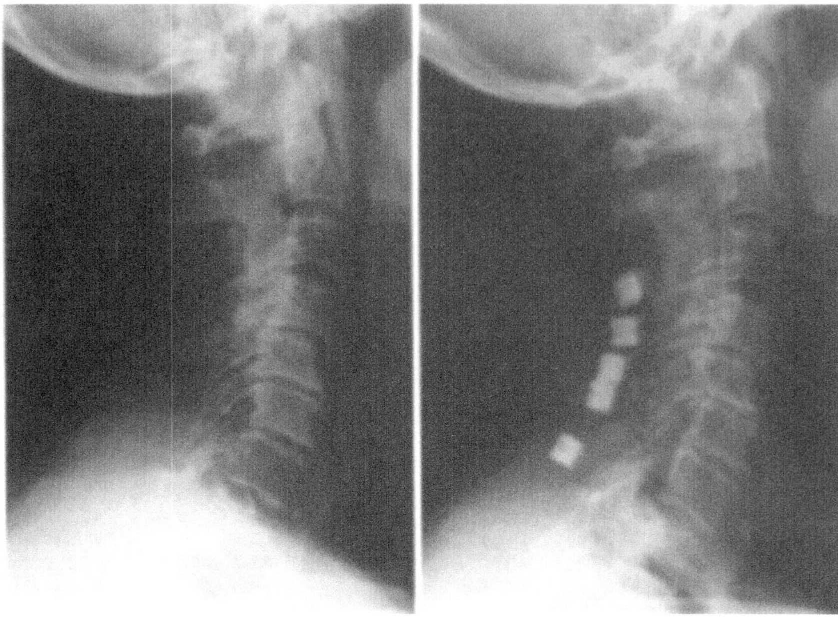

Fig. 3. A 78-year-old man was treated by laminoplasty (Kurokawa method) for cervical spondylotic myelopathy. **a** Preoperative X-ray showing severe spondylotic change in the cervical spine. The patient had complained of preoperative neck pain. **b** Two years after surgery, an X-ray showed no kyphotic deformity of the cervical spine. He continued to complain of neck pain for more than 2 years after surgery

Table 1. Surgical procedure and diagnosis

	n	CSM	OPLL
Kirita-Miyazaki method			
With collar (group A)	43	19	24
Kurokawa method			
With collar (group B)	18	6	12
Without collar (group C)	47	25	22
Total	108	50	58

CSM, cervical spondylotic myelopathy; OPLL, ossification of posterior longitudinal ligament

A, 6 cases in group B, and 3 cases in group C had a severe reduction in cervical ROM.

In patients treated by the Kirita-Miyazaki method, four complained of postoperative axial symptoms. Three of these four cases had preoperative neck pain, one had postoperative kyphotic deformity, and two had a severe reduction in cervical ROM.

Table 2. Risk factors and neck pain persisting for more than 2 years

	Kirita–Miyazaki method (group A)		Kurokawa (with collar) (group B)		Kurokawa (without collar) (group C)	
	n	Postop. axial pain	*n*	Postop. axial pain	*n*	Postop. axial pain
Total number of patients	43	4 (9.4%)	18	2 (11.1%)	47	2 (4.2%)
Preoperative neck pain	13	3 (23.1%)	6	2 (33.3%)	10	2 (20.0%)
Kyphotic deformity	3	1*	0	0	0	0
Severe reduction of cervical ROM	13	2*	6	1*	3	0

ROM, range of motion
* Overlap with preoperative neck pain

In contrast, patients treated by the Kurokawa method with collar fixation after surgery showed no kyphotic deformity, but two cases who had preoperative neck pain complained of axial symptoms, and one had severely reduced ROM of more than 70%. Patients in groups A and B who had preoperative neck pain and postoperative axial symptoms, also showed a reduction in cervical ROM.

In patients treated by the Kurokawa method without collar fixation after surgery, the cases had a severely reduced ROM, but none of them complained of axial symptoms induced by laminoplasty. Another two cases had a residue of the neck pain noticed before surgery. The remaining 42 cases had no axial symptoms postoperatively.

Patients whose preoperative neck pain persisted for more than 2 years after surgery amounted to 23% of group A, 33% of group B, and 20% of Group C.

Discussion

In 1993 and 1996, Hosono et al. [4, 5] described the first investigations of axial symptoms. They compared 72 patients who underwent laminoplasty and 26 patients who underwent anterior interbody fusion. The prevalence of postoperative axial symptoms was significantly higher after laminoplasty than after anterior fusion (60% vs. 19%). In 18 patients (25%) in the laminoplasty group, the chief complaints after surgery were related to axial symptoms for more than 3 months, whereas in the anterior fusion group, no patient reported having such severe pain after surgery. These symptoms were so severe in 13% of the patients that they were given analgesics. They attributed these symptoms to the surgical intervention on the facet joint. It was also reported that 3 out of 4 patients who complained of severe pain persisting for at least 2 years already had that symptom before surgery. These reports are interesting in that the pain experienced by the patients was not induced by laminoplasty, but was a residue of the neck pain they had suffered before undergoing laminoplasty.

In contrast, Kawakami et al. [6] reported that the incidence of axial symptoms was significantly lower in patients after laminoplasty than in patients after anterior decompression and fusion. They considered that the incidence was lower in the laminoplasty group because the duration of external fixation in this group was short enough to prevent muscle atrophy and facet joint contracture, and to maintain a good muscle balance. These findings suggest that the effect of after-treatment, including the duration of external fixation, should be taken into consideration, as well as the surgical stress on the bones, joints, and soft tissue due to posterior surgery.

Kawaguchi et al. [7] compared two groups of patients divided according to the severity of axial symptoms after en bloc laminoplasty. They reported that the surgical procedure was longer and more extensive in patients with severe axial symptoms than in those with mild ones. They also reported that another important factor in relation to axial symptoms is a limited neck ROM. They therefore recommended early mobilization for the maintenance of the neck ROM.

Many authors have considered how to reduce axial symptoms [8–10], but no results have been reported. Our study has shown that postoperative axial symptoms due to kyphosis and/or a reduction in cervical ROM can be decreased by changing the surgical procedure and postoperative management. For patients who complained of pain after laminoplasty, the nature of their pain was a residue of preoperatively existing neck pain. The neck pain remained after surgery in 23% of group A, 33% of group B, and 20% of group C, who all had pain before surgery.

Postoperative axial symptoms resolved within a few months after laminoplasty in the majority of our patients, suggesting that pain in the postoperative recovery period is not a particular disadvantage of laminoplasty. Long-lasting axial symptoms, which are a real problem for patients, are residuals of preoperative neck pain, as was reported by Hosono et al. [4, 5]. Laminoplasty is considered to be less effective for the relief of preoperative neck pain than the anterior procedure, as these may be discogenic pain that needs spinal fusion. It is necessary to identify the cause of preoperative axial symptoms before establishing treatment such as spinal fusion.

Conclusion

We assessed axial symptoms among patients who had had three types of treatment. Four patients treated by the Kirita–Miyazaki method complained of postoperative axial symptoms for more than 2 years. After the change from the Kirita–Miyazaki method to the Kurokara method, no postoperative kyphotic deformity was observed. However, two patients treated by the Kurokawa method with external fixation had persistent axial symptoms. In patients treated by the Kurokawa method without external fixation, no postoperative axial symptoms and no severe reduction in cervical ROM was observed.

Postoperative axial symptoms are unlikely to be a consequence of laminoplasty. The reconstruction of posterior supporting tissue, such as the reattachment of posterior muscles at the time of surgery, as well as early posture exercises, ROM exercises and muscle-strengthening exercises, are key measures in preventing new postoperative axial symptoms. It is important to identify the cause of preoperative axial symptoms, and evaluate the type of pain.

References

1. Yonenobu K, Yamamoto T, Ono K (1998) Laminoplasty for myelopathy. Indications, results, outcome, and complications. In: Clark CR (ed) The cervical spine, 3rd edn. Lippincott-Raven, Philadelphia, pp 849–864
2. Miyazaki K, Kirita Y (1986) Extensive simultaneous multisegment laminectomy for myelopathy due to the ossification of the posterior longitudinal ligament in the cervical lesion. Spine 11:531
3. Kurokawa T, Tsuyama N, Tanaka H, et al. (1982) Enlargement of the spinal canal by the sagittal splitting of the spinous process (in Japanese). Bessatsu Seikeigeka 2:287
4. Hosono N, Yonenobu K, Koizumi M, et al. (1993) Axial symptoms in cervical spondylotic myelopathy (in Japanese). Rinsho Seikei Geka 28:405–411
5. Hosono N, Yonenobu K, Ono K (1996) Neck and shoulder pain after laminoplasty. A noticeable complication. Spine 21:1969–1973
6. Kawakami M, Tamaki T, Iwasaki H, et al. (2000) A comparative study of surgical approaches for cervical compressive myelopathy. Clin Orthop 381:129–136
7. Kawaguchi Y, Matsui H, Ishihara H, et al. (1999) Axial symptoms after en bloc cervical laminoplasty. J Spinal Disord 12:392–395
8. Tsuzuki N, Tanaka H, Iizuka T, et al. (1989) The role of the spinoligamentous complex in the stability of the cervical spine and a method of cervical laminoplasty preserving the spinoligamentous complex (in Japanese). Rinsho Seikei Geka 24:387–396
9. Yonezawa T, Katoh Y, Kitagawa H, et al. (1992) Long-term results of en bloc laminoplasty of the cervical spine (in Japanese). Rinsho Seikei Geka 27:281–286
10. Mochida J, Nomura T, Chiba M, et al. (1999) Modified expansive open-door laminoplasty in cervical myelopathy. J Spinal Disord 12:386–391

Part 6

Perspectives

Future Perspectives of Expansive Laminoplasty

Yoshiaki Toyama

This book has described many diverse techniques for cervical laminoplasty that have been developed and refined in Japan. All members of the Japanese spine community can be proud of this work.

In particular, four prominent spine surgeons, Kirita, Hattori, Hirabayashi, and Kurokawa, deserve special attention. These four individuals, the pioneers of novel techniques, devoted themselves to better patient care, had the ability to gain inspiration from their daily clinical experiences, and had the courage and strength to turn their ideas into reality.

Anterior decompression follow by spinal fusion was the preferred treatment for cervical myelopathy for the majority of surgeons, because it was considered logical to remove anterior pathological structures such as protruded discs, osteophytes, and ossified ligaments anteriorly. However, anterior fusion was not without complications, especially when a lesion involved multiple levels [1]. Analyses of the long-term results of anterior fusion also revealed that recurrent myelopathy due to the development of diseases in adjacent segments was not uncommon, especially in those with spinal canal stenosis [2].

Until the late 1960s, conventional laminectomy, which totally removes the laminae piece by piece along with attached ligamentous structures, had been the standard posterior surgical technique for the treatment of cervical myelopathy caused by multilevel spondylosis and ossification of the posterior longitudinal ligament. However, the surgical results had been rather unpredictable owing to the inherent traumatic nature of laminectomy, and this led to various complications [3, 4].

In 1968, Kirita [5] devised a sophisticated technique in which the laminae were thinned and divided at the midline using a high-speed drill, followed

---

Department of Orthopaedic Surgery, School of Medicine, Keio University, 35 Shinanomachi, Shinjuku-ku, Tokyo 160-8582, Japan

by en-bloc resection of the laminae to achieve simultaneous decompression of the compromised spinal cord. This technique increased the safety of conventional laminectomy and significantly reduced the rate of neurological complications. However, problems such as the vulnerability of the unprotected spinal cord, and the recurrent myelopathy caused by the development of postoperative kyphosis or by the formation of a laminectomy membrane, remained unsolved [6].

To address such problems, Hattori and co-workers [7, 8] devised expansive Z-plasty of the laminae in 1973, in which the laminae were preserved and reconstructed. However, this technique did not gain widespread acceptance because of its demanding technical aspects.

Through their experience with Kirita's method, Hirabayashi et al. [9] refined the technique and devised their own en-bloc laminectomy in which the spinal cord was decompressed by making bony gutters, using a high-speed drill, at the bilateral junctions of laminae and facet joints, followed by simultaneous resection of the whole laminae. This technique ultimately led to the development of expansive open-door laminoplasty by retaining the connection of one gutter as a hinge [10]. Owing to its simplicity and safety, expansive open-door laminoplasty gained the general approval of spinal surgeons who are at the front line of the fight against cervical disease.

Inspired by Hirabayashi's concept of laminoplasty and its favorable long-term results, various modified laminoplasty techniques have been developed. Among these, spinous process splitting laminoplasty, devised by Kurokawa et al. [11], gained popularity because secure reconstruction of the spinal canal could be achieved, thereby providing a protective shell for the decompressed, but still vulnerable, spinal cord, and at the same time restoring stability to the cervical spine.

Both techniques have undergone a variety of refinements and alterations, including the employment of different types of osteotomy, or the use of biocompatible materials and plates, in trying to address the problems of laminar closure and postoperative malalignment [12, 13].

However, it should always be remembered that these two fundamental yet innovative techniques formed the basis for all other procedures, and are still the most viable options for the surgical treatment of compressive myelopathy.

Through continuous efforts to improve and refine the techniques and to establish clear indications, as described in this book, the future of laminoplasty looks promising. However, there still remain a number of questions to be answered and problems to be solved.

The etiology of cervical myelopathy itself still has not been elucidated. The presence of spinal canal stenosis is known to play an important role in the development of myelopathy, and in Japan, the anteroposterior diameter of the spinal canal on lateral view radiographs is routinely used to make the diagnosis of spinal canal stenosis [14]. However, it is not clear whether the Japanese criteria directly apply to all other ethnicities. Moreover, the criteria for evaluating the patient's general, neurological, and psychosocial status, whether preoperative or postoperative, differ in different regions and countries. Universally acceptable criteria for a diagnosis of myelopathy and for spinal canal stenosis, as well as a system to evaluate the treatment outcome accurately, must be established in order to discuss the true efficacy of laminoplasty on a worldwide basis.

The exact mechanism of segmental motor paralysis is another issue that has yet to be clarified, since effective preventive measures have not been established [15]. Even though the preservation of preoperative alignment has been made possible to a certain extent, to date nobody has succeeded in correcting preoperatively established kyphosis to physiological lordosis.

As yet, there is no effective way to regenerate the spinal cord once it is damaged beyond its healing capacity, and the only solution available is to operate on patients with myelopathy before their spinal cord is irreversibly damaged [9].

I hope that many young people who are engaged in the management of cervical myelopathy will be inspired by the articles in this book to find answers to these unsolved problems, and to look for their own "laminoplasty" that would save patients from suffering and disability.

It is a great pleasure to know that our colleagues have developed and refined innovative treatment modalities that have changed the management of cervical myelopathy, one of the most common spinal disorders, and have contributed to improvements in the care of many patients with this disorder. It is our obligation to keep revising the original techniques to improve the outcome, and yet to preserve the fundamental rationale that resides in these original ideas and concepts and pass them on to the next generation.

References

1. Yonenobu K, Fuji T, Ono K, et al. (1985) Choice of surgical treatment for multisegmental cervical spondylotic myelopathy. Spine 10:710–716
2. Toyama Y, Hirabayashi H, Kamata M, et al. (1997) Long-term clinical results of anterior interbody fusion for cervical spondylotic myelopathy. (in Japanese) Higashi Nippon Seikeisaigaigeka Gakkai Zasshi (J East Jpn Orthop Traumatol) 9:487–492
3. Bohlman HH (1977) Cervical spondylosis with moderate to severe myelopathy. Spine 2:151–160
4. Mayfield FH (1976) Complications of laminectomy. Clin Neurosurg 23:435–439
5. Kirita Y (1976) Posterior decompression for cervical spondylosis and OPLL (in Japanese). Shujutsu (Surgery) 30:287–302

6. Cattell HS, Clark GL (1967) Cervical kyphosis and instability following multiple laminectomies in children. J Bone Joint Surg 49A:713–721
7. Kawai S, Sunago K, Doi K, et al. (1988) Cervical laminoplasty (Hattori's method). Procedure and follow-up results. Spine 13:1245–1250
8. Ohyama M, Hattori S, Moriwaki N, et al. (1973) A new method of cervical laminectomy (in Japanese). Chubu Nippon Seikeisaigaigeka Gakkai Zasshi (Central Jpn J Orthop Traumatol) 16:792–794
9. Hirabayashi K, Toyama Y, Chiba K (1999) Expansive laminoplasty for myelopathy in ossification of the longitudinal ligament. Clin Orthop 1359:35–48
10. Hirabayashi K (1978) Expansive open-door laminoplasty for cervical spondylotic myelopathy (in Japanese). Shujutsu (Operation) 32:1159–1163
11. Kurokawa T, Tsuyama N, Tanaka H (1982) Enlargement of the spinal canal by the sagittal splitting of the spinous process (in Japanese). Bessatsu Seikeigeka (Orthop Surg) 2:234–240
12. Itoh T, Tsuji H (1985) Technical improvements and results of laminoplasty for compressive myelopathy in the cervical spine. Spine 10:729–736
13. Matsuzaki H, Hoshino M, Kiuchi T, et al. (1989) Dome-like expansive laminoplasty for the second cervical vertebra. Spine 14:1198–1203
14. Maruiwa H, Chiba K, Watanabe M, et al. (2000) Long-term results of expansive open-door laminoplasty for cervical spondylotic myelopathy (in Japanese). Rinsho Seikeigeka (Clin Orthop Surg) 35:411–416
15. Chiba K, Watanabe M, Maruiwa H, et al. (2000) Segmental motor paralysis after expansive open-door laminoplasty (in Japanese). Rinsho Seikeigeka (Clin Orthop Surg) 35:607–612

Subject Index

GPSR Compliance

The European Union's (EU) General Product Safety Regulation (GPSR) is a set of rules that requires consumer products to be safe and our obligations to ensure this.

If you have any concerns about our products, you can contact us on ProductSafety@springernature.com

In case Publisher is established outside the EU, the EU authorized representative is:

Springer Nature Customer Service Center GmbH
Europaplatz 3
69115 Heidelberg, Germany

Batch number: 10682215

Printed by Printforce, the Netherlands